HELLMUT L

The New Life

Fasting

Guide

Seven Days to a
Healthier, Happier You

INTRODUCTION

PRACTICE

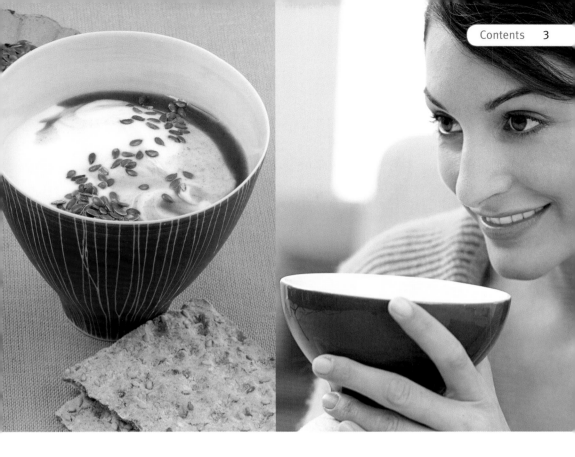

RESOURCES

ABOUT THE AUTHOR

Hellmut Lützner, MD, a specialist in internal medicine, is one of Europe's most experienced fasting doctors. He has supervised fasts for many decades, and he has himself fasted throughout his long life. When he was a child, his parents taught him the art of fasting, and fasting became his focus as a medical doctor as well. For many years Dr. Lützner directed the renowned Kurpark-Klinik at Lake Constance, one of the premier fasting clinics in the world.

Dr. Lützner created this book parallel to an extremely successful TV series on fasting in the late 1970s. It has been updated several times, and continues to be Europe's number one practical fasting guide. Also, this book has since become a basic text used in the education of Fasting Coaches in Germany.

With fasting your quality of life increases, and many illnesses can be halted, even healed. Fasting remains a true adventure in a world where the highest mountain peaks have been climbed and the deepest oceans have been crossed. On a fast, if you are able and willing to travel, you will discover nothing less than the amazing and beautiful landscape of your deepest self, your soul, and a new you will emerge, giving way to a life lived more fully. Have a wonderful journey!

BOOK DISCLAIMER

This book offers a simple, hands-on introduction to the great art of fasting, which is being rediscovered today. Indeed, fasting is a powerful tool when handled wisely. If you are healthy and your medical doctor approves, you can follow this book and discover the ecstatic power of fasting.

However, with growing enthusiasm, there is also a host of misunderstandings and even dangers. Fasting, done unwisely, is perilous and can be fatal. If you are not healthy, if you feel weak for any reason, or if your doctor does not approve, then you **MUST NOT** do this fast. If you are able to fast with your doctor's approval, then you **MUST** follow the guidelines of Dr. Lutzner; especially, you **MUST NOT** interrupt a fast to eat or drink heavily, as this can have serious health consequences.

PLEASE READ THE DISCLAIMER CAREFULLY BEFORE UNDERTAKING ANY FASTING TECHNIQUES DESCRIBED IN THIS BOOK.

By practicing the fasting information presented here, you signify your assent to this disclaimer. If you do not agree to this disclaimer, please do not use the book. The information in this book is presented for the educational and free exchange of ideas and speech in relation to health and wellness only. It is not intended to diagnose any physical or mental condition or function as a substitute for the advice and treatment of a doctor or other licensed professional. **YOU SHOULD CONSULT YOUR PHYSICIAN OR OTHER HEALTH PROFESSIONAL BEFORE STARTING THIS OR ANY OTHER FASTING PROGRAM TO DETERMINE IF IT IS RIGHT FOR YOUR NEEDS. DO NOT START THIS PROGRAM IF YOUR PHYSICIAN OR HEALTH CARE PROVIDER ADVISES AGAINST IT.** In the event that you use any of the information presented here in connection with your own health or diet, the author and publisher of this book assume no responsibility and shall have no liability for any adverse consequence as they are neither legal counselors nor health practitioners and make no claims in this regard.

Persons suffering from anorexia or any other eating disorder should not take part in any fasting activities included in this book and should seek professional medical and psychological attention for these specific needs. We strongly discourage any teenagers from taking part in any fasting activities without first seeking professional medical and psychological counsel.

Certain populations are advised not to fast. Those people include, but are not limited to, pregnant women, nursing mothers, persons with eating disorders, persons with severe anemia, persons suffering obesity, persons with porphyria (genetic metabolic defect), persons suffering from a rare genetic fatty acid deficiency that prevents proper ketosis, persons with heart problems or who have suffered a stroke, persons with mental disorders, persons with kidney or gall bladder stones/issues, persons with magnesium deficiency, or persons suffering from any form of cancer or cancer treatment.

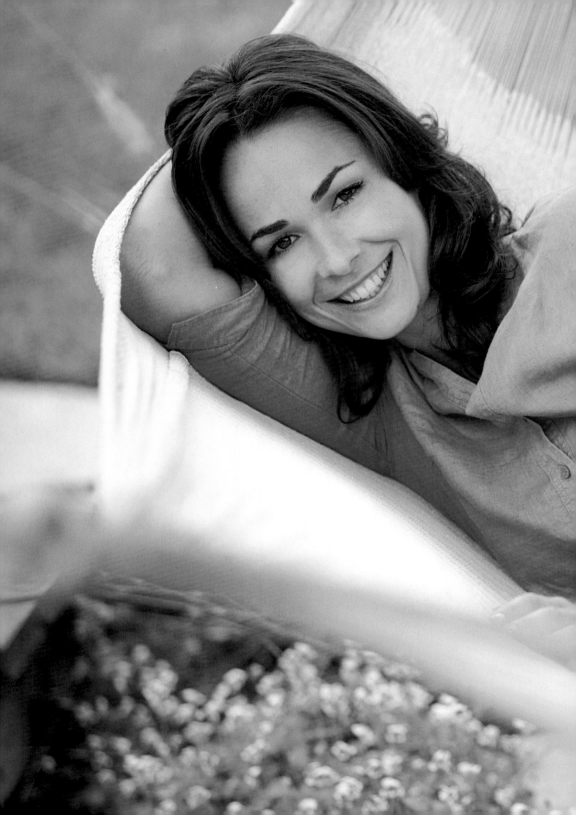

FASTING IS A PART OF LIFE

Stepping back from all the distractions of daily life, finding peace of mind, reflecting on your innermost self—you can do all of this while fasting—and lose weight in the process.

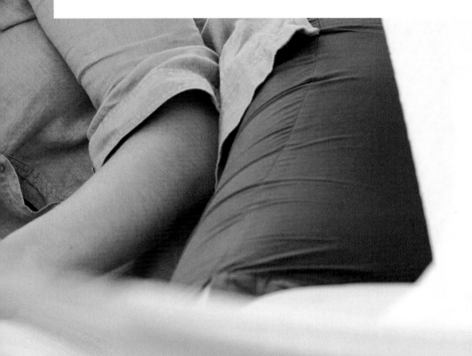

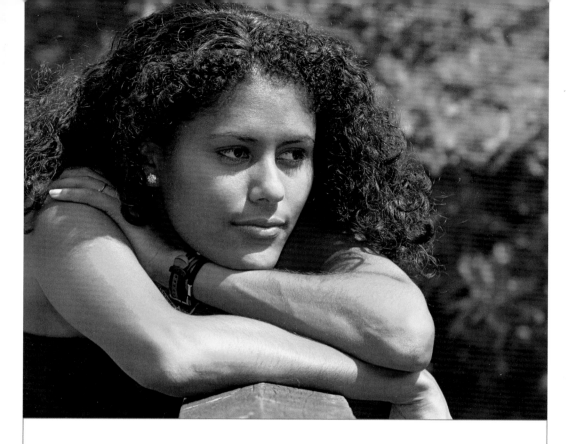

What You Need to Know

Eating and not eating are like waking and sleeping or tension and relaxation—two essential poles that determine a person's life. Eating during the day and fasting at night are part of life's rhythm, so natural that you never even think about it. But if you eat late in the evening, you discover that you have no appetite the next morning: this is your body's signal that the necessary fasting period is not over yet but has just been postponed.

When you are awake during the day, you require 12 to 14 hours of energy to perform all your activities, such as working, or relating to and communicating with the outside world. All types of actions and reactions, as well as the intake of food, are included in these activities. That leaves 10 to 12 hours at night for your metabolism to work its processes (the absorption, conversion, and replenishment of the building blocks of the physical body) and for you to recuperate. The body obtains the energy it needs from its own reserves. During the fasting period at night you are "self-absorbed": you sleep and keep still. Rest, a sense of security, and warmth help you to live on your inner resources. These are the vital foundations for any type of fasting, and you will encounter these concepts time and again in this book.

Fasting during Illness

When you are sick, you also require rest, a sense of security, and warmth—and you want to be left alone more than usual. A feverish child may refuse food and merely ask for cool juice. A sick dog hides in its shelter and eats nothing for days. Ill creatures instinctively behave the right way: they fast. The sick organism requires time for itself and strength to recover. It derives the necessary energy to restore diseased cells and generate healthy cells from the body's own nutritional reserves. Fasting eliminates the effort of digestion, which requires 30 percent of the entire energy output of the organism. The energy freed up by fasting is then used for the work of healing.

GOOD MORNING!
The word *breakfast* actually means "breaking the fast." If you have not fasted during the night, then you do not need "breakfast" in the morning.

This instinctive fasting during a fever or some other illness is a great self-help mechanism from Mother Nature. We know for certain that in people who are otherwise healthy, fever and simultaneous fasting are highly effective aids for healing:

> They exert a strong destructive power on the bacteria that have penetrated your body.
> They inhibit the spread and growth of viruses that may have infected you.
> They strengthen your body's blood and cell defenses.
> They increase your elimination of toxins and other harmful substances.

Fasting and Enhanced Performance

You may already have found that strength, speed, endurance, and mental capacity in no way depend directly on eating. On the contrary, proverbs such as the following tell the real truth: "A fat kitchen makes a lean will." When you have an empty stomach, you actually think better and more quickly. Consider mountain climbers. If they set out at 3 AM, they climb for three, four, or five hours during the extended fasting period before dawn. They do not have breakfast until afterward. The same goes for runners, who will not achieve top performance if they eat before they begin a race.

Even looking at these few examples, it becomes clear that you normally do not live "from hand to mouth." You do not draw your strength directly from food. Instead, your body has its own nutritional reserves. These reserves can be called on more quickly and efficiently than the energy from food, which can be acquired only after the time-intensive and energy-intensive work of digestion. Another phenomenon also refutes the old preconception that you acquire your energy directly from food: you may often feel no desire to eat during or after an exertion requiring strength or endurance. You first satisfy your thirst; only later do you feel hungry.

Athletes, in particular, experience the correlation between performance and fasting more intensely. They know that performance is primarily made possible by energy drawn from the body's own reserves. The fasting metabolism prevents energy losses through the work of digestion and mobilizes the required strength in the most optimal way.

It is possible to live for days, even weeks, without food while achieving astonishing performances. The Swedish doctor Otto Karl Aly reported on an extensive fasting march of 20 Swedes who were convinced that human

The Two Energy Programs of the Body

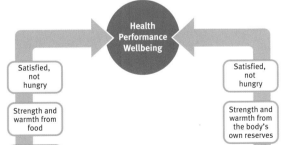

beings could not only live from but also perform well on their body's own reserves. The men marched from Göteborg to Stockholm—310 miles (500 km) in 10 days, or 31 miles (50 km) per day—without consuming any solid food. Each of them required no more than some fruit juice and about 3 quarts of water daily. Dr. Aly reported that, despite their weight losses of 11 to 15½ pounds each, the men still looked great, seemed to be in high spirits, and showed no signs of exhaustion. In fact, they arrived in Stockholm with increased strength and endurance.

Fasting Is a Natural Part of Life

The switch from eating to fasting occurs almost automatically. In fact, these programs run totally by themselves. This is how you can prepare for the proper shift from Energy Program I to Energy Program II (see p. 10):

> By learning about your preprogrammed ability to fast
> By trusting in the safety of this natural approach
> By voluntarily deciding to fast
> By experiencing a thorough evacuation of the bowels, which is the signal from your body to shift and initiate the fast

If you are fasting for the first time, you will discover that your ultimate "yes" to fasting comes during the first few days, when you are surprised to realize that you are not hungry. You will feel good and be productive. This makes it more and more possible for you to come to trust in the body's automatic self-control. Based on the experience that life without food is possible, you will gain an inner assurance that is often admired by those unfamiliar with fasting.

The Signal of Hunger

Hunger is the body's signal, meaning "I am waiting for food. I am prepared to receive food. I produce saliva and digestive juices. My metabolism is switched to Energy Program I."

If the energy from food is absent, this expectation is not fulfilled. The signal of hunger then turns into the feeling called "starving," which ranges from an unpleasant to a tormenting

INTROSPECTION

To discover the times when you are especially healthy, ask yourself the following questions:

> What times do I recall when I was especially fit?
> When was the last time that I ate before I felt fit?
> Did I eat a lot, a little, or perhaps nothing at all?
> Did I use stimulants such as coffee, black tea, cola, nicotine, or alcohol?
> What does "being in my best shape" depend on?

experience: a physical sensation that you can feel gnawing in your stomach and that stubbornly occupies your thoughts. When it is especially bad, your body may respond with dizziness, nausea, and weakness, sometimes accompanied by severely increased sweating and trembling.

A mere glass of fruit or vegetable juice can be enough to eliminate this acute hunger within 5 to 10 minutes. Eating something will have a longer-lasting effect, though, and being full consequently means you have satisfied your physical hunger.

Living on Your "Inner Food"

When you fast properly, you feel no physical hunger, because you have switched to Energy Program II. You are not hungry, because your inner energy source keeps you fully supplied for up to 10 days. As long as you have enough food reserves, you can fast. If you are healthy, your organs work just as reliably and naturally during fasting as in normal everyday life. Perhaps now you can understand why it is often so difficult to skip a meal or simply eat

TIP FOR SUCCESS

Constantly eating too much eventually overwhelms your body's ability to digest. The food remnants left in the intestine trigger the fermentation and decaying processes. The intestine then absorbs the resulting alcohol-like products and directs them into the body. This makes you feel sleepy, ill-tempered, or nervous. You sleep at night as if you have been drugged, or you are restless and cannot fall asleep and stay asleep. To break this vicious cycle, you must regain your balance, purpose, and the joy of eating, as well as recapture your inner peace. Cleanse your bowels thoroughly. Take a break from food by fasting. Get more exercise in fresh air. When you are finished fasting, adjust your diet to the natural rhythm of alternating complete meals with long-lasting satisfaction and breaks from food (see also pp. 92–101).

a bit less—as in a weight-loss diet that allows only 1,000 calories a day. In this situation the body, functioning on Energy Program I, receives too little strength and believes—erroneously—that it is starving. Paradoxically, total abstention from food, meaning life according to Energy Program II, is actually much easier to handle.

Fasting Equals Life without Food

Every person has the capacity to switch to fasting. Fasting simply needs to be experienced and practiced. Naturally, when food is lacking, the body that is accustomed to fasting switches more easily than the untrained body. But even after a single fast it becomes much easier the next time to abstain from food for a certain period.

To a trained body, it is no longer a problem to forgo a meal. Even a neutral position between Energy Program I and Energy Program II can be achieved with little effort. It becomes easier to subsist for a longer period on a weight-reduction diet by covering energy needs partially from food and partially from the body's own reserves—without experiencing hunger. This ability starts to develop during the gradual reintroduction of food after only a week of fasting.

These explanations make it clear that "fasting equals life without food" is a natural part of our existence. So it seems strange that most people are still unfamiliar with this principle. They find it inconceivable that someone could live without food and perhaps also work during this time. They fear deprivation, illness, and even death, and it is amazing how stubbornly these prejudices persist. We need only look at nature, however, to show us the fallacy of this attitude.

Wisdom from the Natural World

For many animals living in the wild, a period of weeks or even months of fasting is part of their normal annual life cycle. This seemingly special ability to adapt is simply a type of survival capability planned by Mother Nature during a time when food is scarce or unavailable. Wolves, for example, can live for days or weeks

VITAMIN DEFICIENCY THROUGH FASTING?
When you are fasting, any additional vitamin and mineral supplements are generally unnecessary. If you are healthy, your body has adequate reserves. In addition, by consuming fruit and vegetable juices or vegetable broth, you can supply the body with organic nutrients every day.

without food and still travel long distances. Like most predators, they feed when food is available. If they cannot find prey they live on their nutritional reserves.

Wild game in high mountainous regions, such as ibexes, chamois, deer, and groundhogs, increase their food intake during the fall until they have accumulated a substantial layer of stored fat. They draw on this store of fat during the hard winter season. While the marmot hibernates (considerably reducing its daily energy requirement), ibexes, chamois, and deer must fight for their survival in the snow and cold. The mating season, characterized by heated battles between rival males and the fertilization of the females, occurs precisely during this fasting period, which should make the point obvious to any skeptic: in no way does fasting reduce vitality. On the contrary, it improves life exponentially.

The Rich Tradition of Human Fasting

Just as for animals today, for people in the past the innate ability to use stored food energy was a biological necessity for survival—even during extremely long periods of food deprivation and even when essential building blocks of the body were partially broken down. The path to starvation is long, and entire peoples would have become extinct without this ability.

Living in Harmony with Nature

The story of the Hunzakut, an ancient civilized people, is a vivid example suggesting that fasting can be more than merely a means of survival. This group of 10,000 to 20,000 people continues to live in a high valley of the Karakoram Mountains north of the Himalaya range, an area that is now part of Pakistan. Until the early 20th century the Hunzakuts had had almost no contact with the outside world. Dr. Ralph Bircher, a Swiss medical writer and economist who studied them, reported amazing things about them. The fields of the high valley did not produce enough to feed people throughout the year, so they had to fast for weeks, sometimes up to two months, until the barley was ripe in June. The

UNBELIEVABLE ENERGY RESERVES
During the second half of the summer, migratory birds eat more than they need: when they fly off to warmer regions, they often weigh twice their normal weight. The reason for the "gluttony" is that with the fuel of fat they manage to make nonstop flights of distances up to 3,100 miles (5,000 km). Following this strenuous performance, their body weight returns to normal.

people remained cheerful and content during this time, performing their work as usual. They labored hard in the fields and rebuilt irrigation channels that had been destroyed by avalanches. They were unfamiliar with the concept of doctors and had no need for police. Their lives followed the cycles of nature.

Today this valley is accessible by the Karakoram Highway from China to Pakistan, through a pass at an elevation of 17,716 feet (5,400 m). Our so-called civilization has free rein to import sugar, white flour, and prepared foods. The people "no longer need to starve," as some Pakistanis put it. But the Hunzakuts continue to recognize the laws inherent in their culture: fasting is the natural time of inner peace, family happiness, and high productivity. The frugal meals that follow the fasting suffice to fulfill all the tasks and obligations required in a mountainous world at an elevation of between 6,562 and 22,966 feet (2,000–7,000 m). For decades the Hunzakuts have continued to rely on their ancient wisdom regarding life and survival.

Living with a Lot—and with a Little

In this day and age we are increasingly surrounded by available food sources, making it difficult for us to understand the deeper meaning of solitary fasting or voluntarily refraining from food. Still, certain indigenous peoples in Australia and Africa continue to adapt to their sparse environments in much the same way as their ancestors did for millennia: they go through periods when they eat from their food reserves, alternating with periods when food is not available.

This continuous alternating between fasting and nonfasting also led to the development of religiously motivated fasting. Fasting is a way for people to thank God for the opportunity to survive and to have enough to eat. The experience of fasting is seen as the path to inner order and is a process of personal development and maturation. The great religious teachers, such as Moses, Christ, Buddha, and Muhammad, attained an understanding of the basic order of human existence during long voluntary periods of fasting. They

FASTING KEEPS YOU YOUNG
Abstaining from food regularly (at least once a year) has a positive effect on aging. Although it might not *prevent* biological aging, it can definitely delay the premature aging processes, because the environmental toxins you increasingly absorb in today's world are eliminated from your body.

were at peace with themselves, concentrating solely on their inner voices, and were not distracted by interruptions such as the consumption of food. This experience led to the insight that only during phases of contemplation can we be truly close to ourselves and to God. But even the church has often failed in the history of fasting: church prescriptions and rules about fasting were not observed and were undermined. People increasingly resisted fasting, often for fear of damaging their health. All that remained of the principles of fasting were rigid, meaningless rules.

Putting It All into Practice

The following section presents a brief checklist about what fasting actually means and what it does *not* mean. A positive attitude toward fasting is half the battle. Do not look at fasting days as periods of self-denial but rather as an asset to your life—as the opportunity to have new and intense experiences.

What Fasting Is

> A natural state of human life
> A state in which your body is capable of living on inner nutrition and internal control
> A practice you can adopt as an independent person who is free to make his or her own decisions
> A practice having an impact on your entire being, on each individual cell of your body, as well as on your soul and your mind
> The best opportunity for you to stay in shape or get back in shape
> A strong impulse to change your (ingrained) lifestyle, if this is necessary

What Fasting Is Not

> Starving (if you are starving, you are not fasting)
> Related to deprivation and scarcity
> Merely eating less
> Abstinence from meat on Friday or following similar rules (that would only be abstention)

EXPERIENCE IT FOR YOURSELF

The time is right for a fresh look at the value of fasting. Nothing is more convincing than feeling and experiencing it for yourself. Fasting needs nothing external—just your own participation.

> A fad promoted by extremists
> Necessarily related to religion (although it may be)

The Benefits of Fasting

Fasting is more than just a quick and pleasant method for getting rid of extra pounds. It has myriad positive effects on the body, mind, and soul. For example, it probably offers the best opportunity for disengaging from the excesses of our consumption-oriented age by (once again) eating mindfully. In addition, fasting is one of the few successful means by which people can detoxify biologically in a polluted environment. Fasting can also help to alleviate dependence on medications and stimulants. At the same time, it

---

THE FIVE BASIC RULES OF FASTING

1. **Eat absolutely no food during the 5 to 10 fasting days—just drink fluids.** Drink unsweetened (herbal) tea, vegetable broth, fruit or vegetable juice, and, of course, water—even more than what is required to quench your thirst.

2. **Avoid everything that is not essential—** anything that has become a favorite habit but that does harm to the body during fasting. This includes taking in substances such as nicotine and alcohol in any form, sweets, coffee, or medications—dispense with as many of these things as you can. Do not use any nonessential medicine such as diuretic pills, appetite suppressants, or laxatives.

3. **Detach from your daily routine.** Spend time away from work and family attachments; from the appointment calendar, telephone, and e-mail; and from magazines, radio, and television. Instead of sensory overload from the outside world, tune in to yourself. Rather than letting yourself be controlled externally, listen to your inner voice and let yourself be guided by it.

4. **Be in harmony with nature.** Do everything your body tells you is good for it. If you are exhausted, sleep until you feel rested. If you like exercise, go hiking or swimming or play sports. Do whatever is fun for you. Go for a stroll, read, dance, enjoy music, and engage in hobbies.

5. **Promote all the ways your body eliminates waste or toxic elements.** Evacuate your bowels regularly, cleanse your kidneys through drinking water, sweat, do breathing work, and take care of your skin.

---

supports the decongestion and elimination of waste products in body tissue, which makes fasters feel free of pain and comfortable. Fasting results in beautiful skin and tight connective tissue.

Fasting helps to preserve physical and mental capacities, especially during menopause in women and the midlife crisis in men.

Fasting has become increasingly important as preventive therapy, because risk factors for a serious illness can often be diagnosed at an early stage (see pp. 99–100).

Therapeutic fasting is even considered the most clinically effective and safest therapy possible for treating nutrition-dependent metabolic diseases. According to Dr. Otto Buchinger, a long fasting treatment is a "royal path of healing" for many acute and chronic illnesses. Physicians who specialize in fasting therapy can confirm this statement, based on their own experiences.

TIP FOR SUCCESS

If you are unsure of how and when to start fasting, simply take advantage of one of the opportunities that are offered almost daily:

> Do not force yourself to eat when you have no appetite. For many people this is especially the case in the morning. The first meal should then be lunch (a morning fasting).
> Fast when you have eaten too much—for example, after holidays or when you have an upset stomach or diarrhea. Fast until a natural sense of hunger develops again. Fast if you have a fever during illnesses such as the flu, the common cold, tonsillitis, or bronchitis.
> Plan a short fast of five days during a week that you anticipate being less stressful. All it takes is some courage and the desire to try something new.

Successful Styles of Fasting

The following examples show that fasting can have many variations. All seven have been practiced successfully.

Fasting the Buchinger Way

Tea or juice fasting, as recommended by Dr. Buchinger, is in my opinion the most suitable form of independent fasting. When you are fasting, drink two cups of herbal tea in the morning and afternoon each. Enjoy vegetable broth for lunch, and have fruit juice or vegetable juice in the evenings. Of course, you should drink lots of water throughout the day and evening.

Raw Juice Fasting (According to Eugen Heun)

In this form of fasting one drinks a glass of freshly squeezed fruit or vegetable juice three to five times a day and at least 2 quarts of water throughout the day and evening.

Whey Fasting

Whey, a dairy product, is an excellent source of protein, minerals, and vitamins. Look for whey in health food stores. Consume 1 quart of whey, distributed throughout the day, supplemented with herbal teas and fresh fruit and vegetable juices. Dietary therapeutic whey is enriched with protein, which is the reason it is primarily recommended for slender people and for the second half of very long fasting periods (to fill up the body's own protein reserves). Drinking whey is better suited for detoxification than consuming the more solid form of milk, because it contains less protein and fewer calories.

Oatmeal Fasting

This form of fasting is especially suitable for people with sensitive stomachs and intestines (find out more on p. 37).

Water Fasting

This is the strictest form of fasting because it completely dispenses with calories and alkaline elements. One is allowed only pure spring or mineral **water:** 1½ quarts daily if you are of average weight or 2 to 3 quarts if you are overweight.

Tea Fasting

In this form of fasting, drink two cups of tea made from various herbs—without honey or other sweeteners—three times per day; only water is permitted in between. Compared with water fasting, tea fasting has the advantage of allowing you to drink warm and alkaline beverages. This is often used as the prelude for the F. X. Mayr therapy.

F. X. Mayr Therapy

A few days of tea fasting are followed by a milk-and-roll diet. The period of abstinence is followed by intensive training in proper chewing.

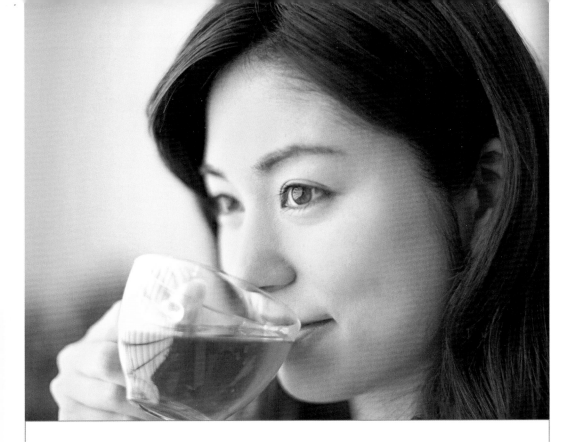

Fasting When You Are Healthy

Should you fast on your own? Yes, if you think you are healthy and physically fit and if you feel confident that you can maintain discipline and have the necessary willpower. Even older people, teenagers 16 or older (with their fasting parents), and disabled persons can fast at home if their bodies function normally. (In theory healthy pregnant and lactating women can also fast, but it is not recommended today, as our communities are polluted with environmental toxins. So long as we do not know whether and how the detoxification process affects an unborn child, fasting should be done only before conception or after the child has been weaned.)

Talk to your doctor before you start. Even if your doctor has had no experience with fasting, he or she can determine the state of your health and discuss the effectiveness of medications during your fast.

What Is the Best Way for You to Fast?

Fasting is easiest to do in a group of like-minded people. If these people happen to be your friends, fasting can be quite exciting. In a fasting community, experiences are multiplied, interpersonal relationships become closer, and members of the group help and support each other. To this end the fasting group should meet regularly to share information and experiences and to plan activities together. Each group member should also have a home of his or her own—in the literal and figurative sense—so that he or she can be alone if desired. An experienced doctor can be consulted for the fasting week. The group should also consider whether a trained fasting coach should give advice and support.

When one is fasting with a partner, the group guidelines apply on a smaller scale: the shared time and the experience of fasting together, your relationship with yourself and your partner, and the mutual help you can provide each other can deepen the partnership. This guideline also applies here: both partners should have the opportunity of retreating into their own space (see p. 69).

It is more difficult to fast alone. Solo fasting requires a considerable degree of discipline and courage, as well as the willpower to abstain and the ability to control yourself. If you have successfully completed the week of fasting on your own, you can be justifiably proud. For the reasons mentioned earlier, however, it

TIP FOR SUCCESS

Do you suffer from osteoarthritis in the fingers, knees, or hips? A fasting therapy under a physician's supervision can significantly reduce the pain. Joint function also improves through abstinence from food, which was demonstrated by a study from the University Hospital of Jena (Germany) in 2007. In some cases the dosage of medication taken for arthritis can be reduced as a result of fasting, even after therapy has ended, because you learn a great deal about proper nutrition during a hospital stay. This allows you to proactively slow the rate at which your joints wear down.

certainly is better if you fast under someone else's guidance the first time. Then you can try fasting alone the next time.

During the fasting week any doctor experienced in fasting can act in a consulting role. In addition you can get extensive advice from trained fasting coaches, who are increasingly available in the United States.

Not only professionals but also any person with experience in fasting can provide help and support to a healthy individual who is fasting for the first time. This is a matter of mutual trust, and the most important aspect is sharing experiences with each other. It is good, and it *feels* good, to be able to fast with understanding. Someone is close by—someone who is familiar with the entire process and available if you need help (also see p. 69).

Where and When Is It Best for You to Fast?

You can fast wherever you feel at ease, where you experience comfort and warmth, and where you have a sense of security. Any place you enjoy, where you can engage in your favorite sport (or just be lazy when you feel like it), is fine. In short, fast in the surroundings that appeal to you the most, where you have peace and can be left alone, and where you are not under stress or pressure. This could be at home, in a hotel or condo on vacation, in the home of a friend, or at a remote mountain cabin. You should also take into consideration that people who are fasting often have the need to withdraw into their proverbial shells.

Fasting at Home

If you want to fast at home, keep in mind that this is where you are most likely to fall prey to all your usual eating and drinking habits. You are living in your familiar space. Above all, you are surrounded by familiar people. Thousands of invisible threads connect each of us with our habitual setting—and unfortunately, this includes the kitchen, refrigerator, pantry, dining table, and liquor cabinet.

The greatest obstacle to fasting at home, however—and this is very important to keep in mind—is the attitudes and

WHAT IS A FASTING CLINIC?

Trained fasting physicians, as well as nurses with one to two years of specialized training, work in a fasting clinic. The types of therapy offered are based on naturopathic treatments. Meals follow a healthy whole-food diet plan. Additional amenities offered by such clinics typically include discussion groups, a teaching kitchen, and a customized exercise program.

prejudices of your relatives and neighbors who may provide you with "good" and unsolicited advice. You might hear people say, "I recently read in the paper that . . . ," or "Go ahead and eat something—I'm sure it won't hurt you," or "You'll starve to death if you keep this up!" And you, the tormented faster, will desperately attempt to escape into solitude and silence. You will quickly learn that, whatever challenges they present, your partner who is cooking the meals or your hungry children returning from school will bother you, the silent faster, a lot less than all the unsolicited advice.

Fasting in Everyday Life

You can also fast while going through your daily routine—which, for many, is divided equally between home and the workplace.

WHEN MUST YOU NOT FAST ON YOUR OWN?

Do not fast on your own if any of the following conditions is true:

> You still have doubts about fasting after reading this book.

> You have been depressed for a long period of time or are emotionally unstable.

> You still feel exhausted after a recent illness or operation.

> You are overwhelmed, nervous, or distraught. Wait until you feel better.

> You are suffering from an eating disorder such as binge eating, anorexia, or bulimia; you should fast only while also undergoing psychotherapeutic treatment.

> You must take medication. In this case you should go to a fasting clinic or fast under the supervision of a fasting physician.

> You are uncertain whether you are actually healthy or not. Get a checkup from your general practitioner and have all risk factors examined. A stay at a fasting clinic would probably be ideal for your initial fast.

> You do not consider yourself healthy: for example, if your blood pressure is too low or too high, if you have been diagnosed with cancer, or if you are considerably overweight (see p. 99). If this is the case, you should not fast without the advice of a doctor who is experienced in fasting. Please carefully read the chapter on Therapeutic Fasting.

A number of people regularly fast in this way, and they often report that the activity in their everyday lives greatly distracts them from thinking about eating. Despite this useful distraction, though, fasting while working requires a good deal of discipline and inner strength. If you fast while carrying on your everyday life, you should be aware that it is a more difficult form of fasting. If you have already experienced some form of fasting, however, you probably already know whether you can handle this. Apart from the many temptations you will face and the challenges your colleagues may present, there are other risks you need to be warned about:

> Your "inner speed" slows down during fasting; everything takes longer.
> Your cardiovascular system is not as stable during fasting. This is commonly the case for only a few hours a day, but what will you do if things become stressful right when it matters?
> You may become more emotionally sensitive, which translates into your having lower defenses and less protection against ugly emotional attacks and injustices.
> If you must drive, you should exercise caution, as your ability to respond and to concentrate on the road can be reduced while fasting.

Fasting on Vacation

No doubt a vacation or a guided fasting week is a better alternative for your initial fasting experience. Plan your week of fasting in advance. The ideal situation is to take time off from work. If this is not possible, then at least try to schedule the fasting week during a time when you are not feeling especially pressured and can steer clear of social obligations.

Fasting and being unencumbered belong together. This means being free of the compulsions and obligations of a strenuous daily life—free from a hectic pace, noise, and unpleasant smells in the air. The most likely scenario for achieving this is when you are on vacation or together with people who share your outlook. If

FASTING WITH THE RHYTHM OF THE YEAR

Discover for yourself which season is most conducive for you to fast. In the spring, when everything outside grows and thrives, people usually have a strong desire to renew themselves. Many folks tend to have less of an appetite in the summer and find it easy to drink fluids in those months. The mood of autumn invites a deeper look at our own lives. Winter is an ideal time to fast for those who perspire a lot and often feel hot.

you like to be active, you could plan a hiking fast, which combines fasting with bicycling, mountain climbing, sailing, swimming, dancing, or enjoying a sauna. If you prefer to spend your time in contemplation, there are also fasting weeks with opportunities for a retreat such as staying at a monastery, engaging in yoga and meditation, exploring nature, or combining fasting with a number of wellness activities or various forms of creative expression.

The Fasting Week for Healthy People

In some areas fasting weeks for healthy persons are organized in the form of courses and under the direction of fasting coaches. These are highly recommended for first-time fasters because of the comprehensive information and supportive fasting community they provide. Fasting weeks simultaneously serve the purpose of continuing education and self-realization. The various supplementary programs improve one's quality of life: a stronger sense of your body, creativity, learning how to eat consciously, relaxation, meditation, self-help from Mother Nature's pharmacy, and much more. Please note that a fasting week for healthy people is *not* therapeutic fasting; that would require the preconditions described starting on page 104.

Almost Ready

As a first-time faster, you should not plan to fast for more than the week suggested in this guide: one day for preparation, five days for fasting, and at least two days for breaking the fast and building up the diet. The Fasting Week at a Glance (see pp. 26–29) is a guide to help you find the right information quickly whenever necessary.

It can be best to begin your fasting week on a Saturday. Then you have a full week ahead of you, during which you should only have to take care of yourself. If it is your second or third time fasting—provided you are healthy and feel well—you can fast for up to 10 days. Longer fasts, however, will require more days to reacclimate. Breaking the fast and building up the diet require just as much care and attention as fasting itself.

IMPORTANT
In no case should you fast during a work week if any of the following conditions is true:

> You work in a job that is unusually challenging.

> You are responsible for the well-being of others in your job.

> You must operate machines and consequently are at risk for accidents. This includes professions such as lathe operator, taxi or bus driver, crane operator, roofer, or pilot.

Take a fasting vacation. Experienced fasters know that it is best to fast while on vacation. The nervous system switches from the struggle for existence to recuperation—an important precondition for proper fasting and the best guarantee that the fasting will be successful.

Preparation Day

Food Intake
Morning: Fruit and nuts or Bircher muesli (see p. 84 for recipe)
Noon: Raw vegetable plate (see p. 84 for recipe), boiled potatoes, cooked carrots, and preferably organic yogurt with sea buckthorn and flaxseed (see p. 82 for recipe)
Afternoon: 1 apple and 10 hazelnuts
Evening: Fruit or fruit salad (with flaxseed or wheat bran), 1 cup plain yogurt, preferably organic, and flatbread; drink plenty of fluids

Elimination
Soften intestinal contents by making sure there is enough dietary fiber in your food. Take flaxseed or wheat bran. Drink plenty of fluids.

Exercise and Rest
Run or go for a walk, enjoy fresh air, and let yourself rest.

Body Care
Take a bath, put on fresh underwear, and relax.

Awareness
Be mindful; detach yourself from your everyday routine.

First Day of Fasting

Food Intake
Morning: Herbal tea, Glauber's salt (sodium sulfate decahydrate) with lemon, diluted in water as per the directions on the package. On the side have a strong sweetened peppermint tea for taste
Late morning: More water or tea
Noon: Vegetable broth (see recipes, pp. 35–36)
Afternoon: Tea with ½ teaspoon honey
Evening: Fruit and vegetable juice or vegetable broth

Elimination
Morning: Evacuate your bowels thoroughly.
Noon: The liver detoxifies better when you are lying down.

Exercise and Rest
Morning: Sleep in, exercise, stay home.
Noon: Rest and take a short walk.
Evening: Go to bed early.

Body Care
Morning: Keep your feet warm.
Noon: Keep your body warm; use a liver compress (see p. 52).

Awareness
Morning: Letting go rather than taking in.
Noon: Enjoy the comfort of warmth.

Second Day of Fasting

Food Intake
Morning: Herbal tea with ½ teaspoon honey
Late morning: Water occasionally
Noon: Vegetable broth (see recipes beginning on p. 35)
Afternoon: Fruit tea or herbal tea with ½ teaspoon honey
Evening: Fruit juice, vegetable juice, or vegetable broth (see pp. 35–36 for recipes)

Elimination
Morning: Cleanse kidneys and tissues. Drink more than usual.
Noon: Is your urine light in color? If not, then drink more.

Exercise and Rest
Morning: Stretch, do yoga, go for a walk.
Noon: Take a nap.
Afternoon: Go on a brisk walk.

Body Care
Morning: Use cold water to invigorate your face; rub down your skin, and when possible expose it to fresh air.
Noon: Keep your body warm, use a liver compress (see p. 52), and warm your hands and feet. Do not take a full bath or use the sauna.

Awareness
Allow yourself to be tired, let go, and feel the freedom from hunger.

Third Day of Fasting

Food Intake
Morning: Herbal tea with ½ teaspoon honey
Late morning: Water occasionally
Noon: Tomato broth (see p. 36 for recipe)
Afternoon: Fruit tea or herbal tea
Evening: Fruit juice, vegetable juice, or vegetable broth (see pp. 35–36 for recipes)

Elimination
Morning: Evacuate your bowels. Perform an enema at least every other day, starting today (if necessary, take Epsom salts as well).
Late morning: Stimulate bowel movements gently with whey or sauerkraut juice.

Exercise and Rest
Exercise or go for a walk, but all in moderation. Take a nap. Create a rhythm for the nights; if you are unable to sleep, use the time mindfully.

Body Care
Morning: Take a shower, alternating hot and cold water, and then scrub and oil your skin, preferably with a natural body oil.
Noon: Keep your body warm and use a liver compress (see p. 52).

Awareness
Awaken your vital **forces:** "What does my body need?" "What is my soul hungry for?"

Fourth Day of Fasting

Food Intake
Morning: Herbal tea with ½ teaspoon honey
Late morning: Water occasionally
Noon: Carrot broth (see p. 36 for recipe)
Afternoon: Fruit tea or herbal tea
Evening: Fruit juice or vegetable juice

Elimination
Are your bowel movements spontaneous, without use of a laxative? (This is rare.) Is your urine light in color? If not, drink more. Offensive-smelling perspiration and breath are normal. Peppermint tea helps.

Exercise and Rest
Be active and hike. Engage in sports and physical work, alternating with rest and relaxation.

Body Care
Walk barefoot in the dew or run in the snow. Sweat, shower, oil your skin, and lie down to relax. You should be strong enough for the sauna or a full bath (plan to rest afterward).

Awareness
Morning: Enjoy the fresh morning air. Exercise gives you a sense of satisfaction and contentment.
Noon: Notice the pleasant warmth you feel in your well-exercised limbs.

Fifth Day of Fasting

Food Intake
Morning: Herbal tea
Late morning: Water occasionally
Noon: Celery broth (see p. 35 for recipe)
Afternoon: Fruit tea or herbal tea
Evening: Fruit juice, vegetable juice, or vegetable broth (see pp. 35–36 for recipes)

Elimination
Morning: Cleanse bowels with an enema (if necessary, take Epsom salts). Whey or sauerkraut juice gently stimulates bowel movements.

Exercise and Rest
Fill your need for exercise, but adapt to your fasting condition. Instead of ignoring obstacles, accept them.

Body Care
Morning: Scrub, shower, and oil your skin.
Noon: Warm your feet and use a liver compress (see p. 52).
Evening: Prepare for the night and use natural sleep aids (e.g., hop tea, relaxation, or autogenic training).

Awareness
Today you will shop for food that you will build up gradually. Be proud of yourself, and happy that you can go food shopping without feeling the urge to buy too much.

First Build-Up Day

Food Intake
Morning: Herbal tea
Late **morning:** Break the fast with a very ripe (or steamed) apple.
Noon: Potato vegetable soup (see p. 79 for recipe)
Afternoon: Continue to drink as before.
Evening: Tomato soup (see p. 80 for recipe), buttermilk with flaxseed, flatbread, and soaked dried fruit

Elimination
Morning: Carefully reaccustom your body to taking in food. Elimination is still important. Fill your intestine with bulky foods. Drink plenty of liquids.

Exercise and Rest
Exercise or go for a walk *before* breaking the fast; rest at noon; and take it easy.

Body Care
Morning: Use Sebastian Kneipp's regimen of cold stimuli (see p. 45) to awaken your life force.
Noon: Lie down once a day. Use a liver compress (see p. 52). Apply a Priessnitz body compress if you have an unpleasant sensation of fullness (see p. 56).

Awareness
Today the focus is on eating: **less is more.**

Second Build-Up Day

Food Intake
Morning: Morning drink, dried fruit, and cracked wheat soup (see p. 81 for recipe)
Late **morning:** Water occasionally
Noon: Leaf salad, boiled potatoes, cooked carrots, and organic yogurt with sea buckthorn (see pp. 81–82 for recipes)
Afternoon: Herbal tea
Evening: Raw carrots, grain vegetable soup, buttermilk with flaxseed, and flatbread (see p. 83 for recipes)

Elimination
Weight gain is normal. Are your bowel movements spontaneous? Take flaxseed and drink liquids. For an unsuccessful urge to empty your bowels, try a half enema or wait for the next dietary build-up day.

Exercise and Rest
Accept down times. Go for a walk; either rest or take a walk after you eat. Avoid exertion.

Body Care
Morning: Scrub skin, get fresh air, and take a shower, alternating hot and cold water.

Awareness
Satisfied? Full? Are you content and satiated after your fast?

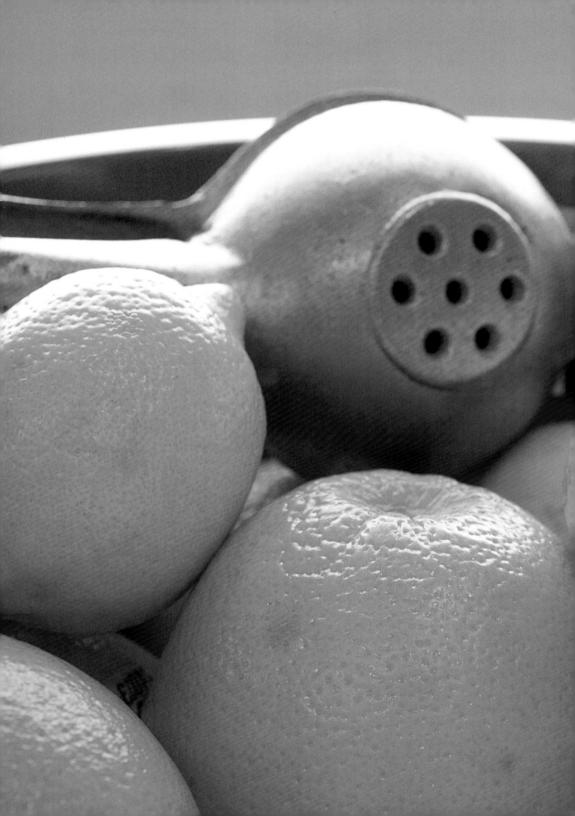

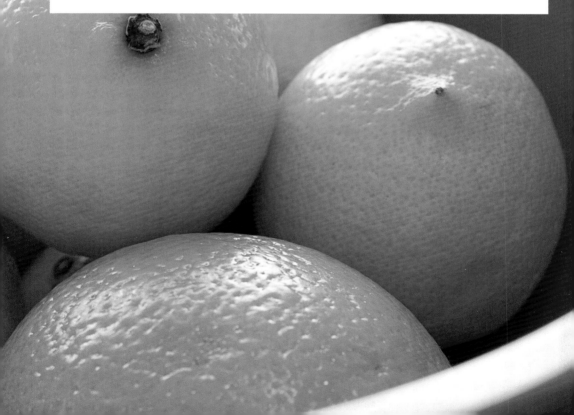

INDEPENDENT FASTING

Fasting does not mean starvation, and it has nothing to do with depriving yourself. Even during the first days of a fast, your body makes the switch and draws energy from its own reserves.

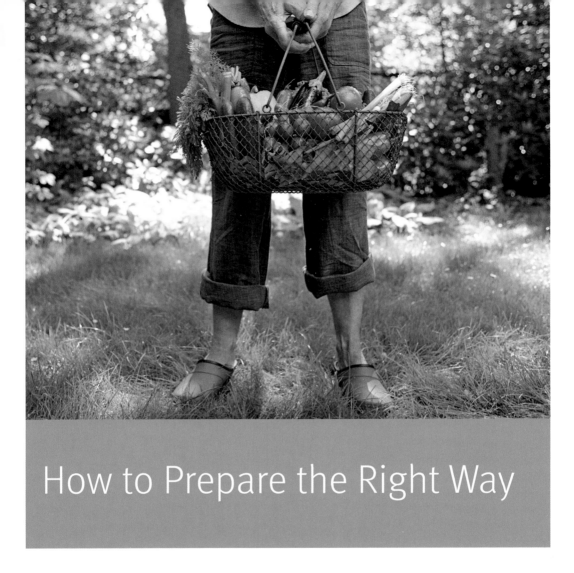

How to Prepare the Right Way

Before a fast you should "clear the decks." Take care of all burdensome chores and pending obligations. Cancel engagements that could cause stress and anxiety. If that is not possible, at least postpone them until a few days after you have completed your fast. To ensure that you can start your fast with a free spirit in the truest sense of the word, nothing (and no one) should impose any burdens on you.

Time to Get Serious

You should have the following items on hand for your weeklong fast:

> Clothing that is somewhat warmer than usual
> An adequate supply of underwear, because in the coming days you will change it more frequently than usual
> Sports clothing and sporting equipment
> Hot-water bottle
> Enema bag (irrigator) with a 12-inch (30 cm) rectal tube (from the drugstore or the Internet)
> Body oil (an organic product if possible)
> Dry natural-bristle brush or loofah glove
> Linen towel

Shopping List

You will need the following foods or beverages for the first six days:

> At least ten 16-ounce bottles of noncarbonated mineral water, unless you have good-quality spring water or tap water available.
> Several varieties of herbal tea. Loose teas or herbs fresh from the garden or farmer's market (e.g., peppermint, lemon balm, verbena) are better than tea bags.
> Vegetables and spices for vegetable broth (recipes are on pp. 35–36).
> Fruit juices (an assortment of your favorites), organic if possible (one large 1½ qt. [1.5 L] bottle or five small 10-oz. [0.3 L] bottles).
> Vegetable juices, likewise organic if possible (one large 1½ qt. [1.5 L] bottle or five small 10-oz. [0.3 L] bottles). Here, too, make sure that you choose a variety you like.
> Sauerkraut juice, one small bottle (if needed).
> Five to 10 whole organic lemons.
> Glauber's salt (sodium sulfate—coarse grain) from the drugstore in 0.5-, 1.0-, or 1.5-ounce (20, 30, or 40 g) packages. Important: Be sure to read page 41 before use.
> Three pounds (1.5 kg) of fruit for the "fruit day," or raw vegetables for the "raw veggie day." If you are planning a "rice day," you will need 6 ounces (150 g) of brown rice (instructions and recipes on the next page).

DON'T WORRY!
Eat and drink as usual on the days before your week of fasting, but do not stuff yourself one last time. Why would you want to? Are you anxious, perhaps? Give away all your remaining prepared food, and stow nonperishable items in a locked cupboard. (Just in case, give the key to a friend to keep for you!)

Recipes for the Preparation Day

On your Preparation Day you can eat all the foods listed in the overview, "Your Fasting Week at a Glance" (see pp. 26–29). You can also implement your Preparation Day somewhat more radically, however. The three stricter regimens that follow are especially intended for people who are overweight. These regimens also show how to lose 2 to 3 pounds (1 to 1.5 kg) quickly and how to lower elevated blood pressure even after your fast is over. (Many people even swear by regularly incorporating a once-a-week Preparation Day into their normal weekly routines.)

The following rule applies every day: drink plenty of mineral or tap water, as well as herbal tea without sugar.

Fruit Day

In this version, over the course of three meals throughout the day eat a total of 3.3 pounds (1.5 kg) of fruit. Be sure not to eat too many bananas, as this sweet fruit can cause constipation for some people. Aim for a healthy mix of a variety of seasonal fruits, including berries. Remember that it is important to chew thoroughly.

Rice Day

On Rice Day eat three 2-ounce (50 g) portions of brown rice, cooked in plenty of water, without salt. In the morning and evening mix the rice with stewed apples or unsweetened applesauce. For lunch, flavor the rice with two stewed tomatoes and chopped herbs.

Fresh Food Day

On Fresh Food Day you eat fruit, fruit salad, or Bircher muesli in the morning, and at noon and in the evening a plate of mixed raw vegetables: leafy greens, grated root vegetables, and sauerkraut. Naturally, you do not prepare the dressing with mayonnaise; instead use a little oil, lemon juice, and spices.

VARIETY IS THE SPICE OF LIFE

Put off shopping for your dietary build-up days until the last day of your fast. You will see how much fun it is to go food shopping during a fast, because now you are much more conscious in your approach to groceries. Moreover, shopping intensifies your anticipation of the first day that you can eat again.

Recipes for Tasty Drinks

Warm vegetable broth is a good source of strength during a fast, not only because it warms you from the inside, but also because it provides necessary vitamins and minerals. Choose among the following four recipes those that you like best, or else vary your choice from day to day.

Potato Broth

8 oz. (250 g) potatoes | 2 carrots | 1/2 stalk of leek | some parsley root if available | 1/4 celery root (celeriac) | 1/2 teaspoon caraway seeds | 1/2 teaspoon marjoram | 1 pinch sea salt | granulated vegetable bouillon | 1 pinch freshly ground nutmeg | 2 teaspoons yeast flakes | 4 teaspoons freshly chopped parsley

1 Thoroughly scrub potatoes, carrots, leek, parsley root, and celery root, but do not peel; cut into small pieces.
2 In a large pot, boil 1 quart water. Cover and boil vegetables together with the caraway seed and marjoram for 10 to 20 minutes or until soft. (If using a pressure cooker, reduce the cooking time to 5 to 7 minutes.)
3 Remove from heat. Pour the soup through a fine sieve, forcing the vegetables through with a wooden spoon. Season to taste with the remaining salt and spices. Sprinkle with yeast flakes and chopped parsley.

Celery Broth

8 oz. (250 g) celery root | a bit of leek and carrots | 1/2 teaspoon caraway seed | 1/2 teaspoon marjoram | granulated vegetable bouillon | 1 pinch freshly ground nutmeg | 2 teaspoons yeast flakes | 4 teaspoons freshly chopped parsley

1 Scrub, wash, and dice celery, leeks, and carrots unpeeled. Boil 1 quart (1 L) water; add vegetables and boil for 10 to 20 minutes or until soft. (If using a pressure cooker, reduce the cooking time to 5 to 7 minutes.)

IMPORTANT
All broth recipes yield four servings.

TIP
You can also season the potato broth with freshly chopped herbs, such as dill, basil, or lovage.

2 Remove soup from heat, force it through a fine sieve, and season to taste with the bouillon and spices. Sprinkle with yeast flakes and chopped parsley.

Tomato Broth

1 lb. (500 g) tomatoes | 1 clove of garlic | a bit of leek, celery, and carrots | 1 pinch sea salt | granulated vegetable bouillon | 1 pinch freshly ground nutmeg | 2 teaspoons oregano or marjoram | 2 teaspoons yeast flakes

1 Wash tomatoes and dice them, cutting out the stem bases. Peel the garlic clove and chop it finely. Wash the remaining vegetables and dice them unpeeled.
2 Boil 1 quart (1 L) water in a pot and cook the prepared ingredients for 10 to 20 minutes or until they are soft (5 to 7 minutes in the pressure cooker).
3 Press the soup through a fine sieve and season to taste with the salt, bouillon, and spices. Sprinkle with the yeast flakes.

TIP
You can further season the tomato broth to taste with a bit of tomato paste.

For a change of pace, when it is very hot in the summer, you can serve the soup—in this case carrot broth—chilled.

Carrot Broth

8 oz. (250 g) carrots | 1/2 stalk of leek | some parsley root and celery | 1 pinch sea salt | granulated vegetable bouillon | 1 pinch freshly ground nutmeg | 2 teaspoons yeast flakes | 4 teaspoons freshly chopped parsley

1 Clean, wash, and chop the unpeeled vegetables into small pieces. Place in a pot with 1 quart (1 L) boiling water. Cook for 10 to 20 minutes (5 to 7 minutes in the pressure cooker).
2 Press the soup through a fine sieve and season to taste with the salt, bouillon, and spices. Sprinkle with the yeast flakes and chopped parsley.

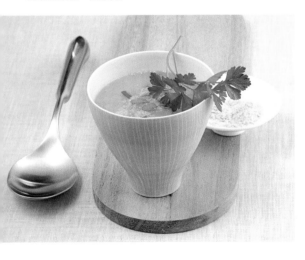

Recipes for Soothing Your Stomach

For people who have sensitive stomachs or sensitive intestinal tracts, or both, it is recommended to fast using the following porridge dishes, because they are particularly easy on the stomach. They can be seasoned to taste with a little sea salt, yeast extract, honey, fruit juice, or vegetable juice.

In cases of acute stomach troubles a sip of thin porridge often helps, even at night or early in the morning. If you are frequently plagued by pain, it is a good idea to fill a thermos bottle with porridge in the evening and keep it by your bedside.

IMPORTANT
Porridge recipes yield one portion each.

Oatmeal Porridge

3 tablespoons oatmeal | 1 pint (0.5 L) water

1   Bring water to a rapid boil, stir in oatmeal, and boil for 5 minutes.
2   Remove from heat. Force the contents through a sieve, and drink the porridge one sip at a time.

Rice Porridge

3 tablespoons rice | 1 pint (0.5 L) water

1   Bring rice to a boil in 1 pint (0.5 L) unsalted water. Cook over low heat until soft, approximately 20 minutes (depending on rice variety).
2   Remove from heat and force the contents through a sieve. While the porridge is still warm, drink it in small sips.

Flaxseed Porridge

½–1 oz. (15–20 g) ground flaxseeds | 1 pint (0.5 L) water

1   Bring flaxseeds to a boil in 1 pint (0.5 L) water. Use a deep pot, as flaxseed boils over easily. Cover pot and cook over medium heat for 5 minutes.
2   Remove from heat and let stand for a few minutes, then skim the porridge and drink in sips.

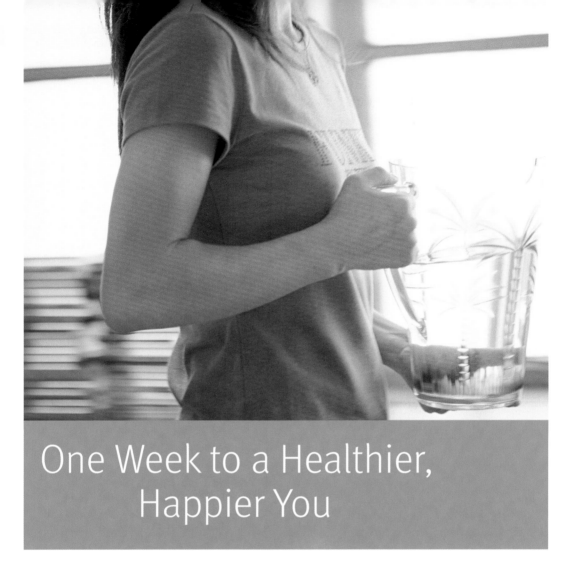

One Week to a Healthier, Happier You

Unburdening means freeing yourself from everything superfluous, both in terms of diet and in psychological or spiritual terms. Remember, this week you are the most important person, and you should be completely there for yourself. Unfinished assignments and chores could easily destroy your inner harmony.

The Preparation Day gets you ready for a week of fasting. While it prepares your body for the transition to abstaining from food, its primary purpose is psychological.

The Preparation Day

> Eat simply and very little—just enough to make you feel satisfied. Eat lots of raw vegetables or fruit. Some people find it beneficial to eat 1 tablespoon of flaxseed three times over the course of the day, preferably mixed with plain, natural yogurt or applesauce. The flaxseeds swell in the intestine, and their fine mucilage can bind to the contaminants and toxins deposited there.

> Preparation also means divesting yourself of your emotional burdens, reducing stress and hectic behavior, letting go of tensions, and awakening to your inner self. If you fast during your vacation, use the Preparation Day to really "arrive." Make yourself at home, go for a stroll, or get a really good night's sleep. Entering into your fast will be much more successful after a day of relaxation than if you try to force your overstressed body to make the transition immediately, without any preparation.

> Say good-bye to cigarettes, alcohol, coffee, and sweets—unemotionally and resolutely: "So long! See you next week!"

> Learn everything about the subject of fasting that you would still like to know. Read more about it, or make contact with people who have fasting experience.

> Start your "Fasting Diary" this very day (see box on p. 59). The inner transition from eating to fasting has already begun.

A FEW THOUGHTS TO GET YOU IN THE SPIRIT

> "I myself have made the decision to fast; I know that I can do it."

> "I have left the stress and confusion of daily life behind me."

> "Finally I have time for myself. Here I am safe and secure; I feel good here."

> "Everything I need is here: a warm home, juice, water, and the well-filled pantry within me. I do not need to worry about anything."

> "I am curious where this journey will lead. I made this decision voluntarily, and I am confident that it will be a good journey. Mother Nature is my guide; I can depend on her."

You May Drink the Following

Morning: 2 cups of herbal tea (chamomile, mallow, rosemary, or lemon balm). If you do not like tea, drink hot unsweetened lemon water.

Late morning: Plenty of water or mineral water. Occasionally suck on a wedge of lemon.

Noon: ½ pint (0.25 L) vegetable broth, prepared by you according to one of the four recipes on pages 35–36. Alternatively, drink fresh vegetable juice diluted with enough water to make ½ pint (0.25 L), or canned or bottled vegetable juice generously diluted with water. You can drink soup or juice, cold or hot, whichever you prefer.

Afternoon: 2 cups fruit tea (rose hip, fennel, or apple peel), with lemon or ½ teaspoon honey or both.

Evening: ½ pint (0.25 L) fruit juice diluted with mineral water to taste, cold or warm as you prefer. Alternatively, vegetable juice or vegetable broth (see Noon).

How to Drink Your Beverages

> Beverages used while fasting provide vitamins and minerals, alkalinity, and easily accessible carbohydrates that compensate for fasting acidosis (overacidification associated with fasting). Drink all beverages one sip at a time. "Chew" every swallow—that is, warm it up or cool it off in your mouth. Savor every drop; drink slowly.

> Between your "meals," be sure to drink additional water or mineral water. It is better to drink more than your thirst requires rather than too little. During a fast, water is an important solvent and "rinse" for the detoxifying body.

> Pure vegetable and fruit juices are too concentrated. For this reason they are best diluted 1:1 with water. If juices do not agree with you, stir in 1 teaspoon flaxseed; the fine mucilage of the flaxseeds will bind aggressive fruit and vegetable acids.

IMPORTANT

Soft drinks of all kinds are as unsuited to fasting as so-called fruit juice beverages, because they all contain large quantities of sugar, increase the blood sugar level, and supply the body with many unnecessary calories.

The First Day of Fasting

Fasting begins with a thorough cleansing of the intestines. The body switches from "intake" to "elimination." Nourishment from within commences; hunger disappears. You are now living from your body's own resources.

During this initial day of fasting it is best to remain at home. Lie down when you feel like it, read, take it easy, or listen to music. In the afternoon take a short walk, but do not undertake anything too strenuous. Avoid taking a hot bath or going to the sauna.

Evacuating the Intestines

Experience shows that commencing the fast is most successful if the intestines are thoroughly evacuated. If, in general, you have healthy bowel habits, you will need only minor assistance: in the morning simply drink a glass (½ cup, or 125 mL) of sauerkraut juice, whey, or buttermilk. This promotes rapid evacuation of the intestines.

More than 4 million Americans have frequent constipation, however. If you fall into this group, you will need additional help. In this case you can encourage the loosening of your bowels in the following ways:

> People of normal weight should dissolve 1 oz. (30 g) of Glauber's salt (sodium sulfate decahydrate) in 14 oz. (400 mL) boiling water. Add 12 oz. (350 mL) cold water and a splash of lemon juice to improve the taste. Drink the liquid one sip at a time.
> People who are overweight and all who tend to suffer from constipation should dissolve 1.5 oz. (40 g) of Glauber's salt (sodium sulfate) in the same amount of liquid.
> People with "brisk" digestion need only dissolve 0.5 oz. (20 g) of Glauber's salt (sodium sulfate) in the same amount of water.

Drink the solution within 15 minutes, but be sure to allow yourself several sips of peppermint tea before, during, and after drinking it to get rid of the salty taste as quickly as possible.

During the next one to three hours you will experience several diarrhea-like bowel movements, which for some people might even continue into the afternoon. Because of this, do not plan anything for this day, and stay near a bathroom.

IMPORTANT

If you have a sensitive gastrointestinal system or tend to have abdominal pain frequently, avoid Glauber's salt (sodium sulfate). This also applies if you are lean or very slender. Instead, take a daily enema (see pp. 46–47), which is just as effective but gentler on the body.

Other Things to Note

If you should experience stomachaches on the first day, go to bed with a hot water bottle on your stomach. Also make sure to keep your feet nice and warm—a hot water bottle can help here, too. Quench your thirst with ample amounts of peppermint tea or water.

Women who take oral contraceptives in the morning should wait up to three hours after the Glauber's salt (sodium sulfate) treatment before taking their pill. This precautionary measure is necessary because the effect of Glauber's salt is to empty the stomach prematurely, in which case the medication will not take effect. If an enema is used, there is no need to delay taking the pill.

The Second Day of Fasting

Occasionally, on the second day of a fast the body is still undergoing transitional changes. As a result, you might experience the following physical effects:

> *Feelings of hunger.* You may feel downright gnawing hunger pangs. Half a glass of water will banish them rather quickly. Under no circumstances should you take an appetite suppressant of any kind.

> *Dizziness and feelings of nausea.* Your body might not yet have adjusted to the typical drop in blood pressure. Feelings of queasiness or occasional episodes of lightheadedness are harmless and will soon pass. (Wormwood tea is helpful in combating these symptoms; see also pp. 58–61.) A walk in fresh air and splashing cold water on your face may also bring quick relief. If the dizziness is too severe, you may want to lie down for a little while. In any event, you should drink plenty of fluids.

> *Headaches, aching limbs, and lower back pain.* These are not uncommon at the beginning of a week of fasting because the dehydration of overly tense and toxin-laden muscles can cause aches, pains, and restlessness. Moist hot compresses, such as a small bag filled with mashed potatoes and applied to the neck, lower back, or afflicted joint, can provide quick relief. A cold wet Priessnitz compress (see p. 56) can also alleviate these symptoms. An enema (see pp. 46–47) or a footbath that gradually increases in temperature (see p. 57) is likewise an effective remedy.

IF YOU ARE OVERCOME WITH HUNGER

Should you still be struggling with feelings of hunger, purge yourself thoroughly with another enema, or drink half a glass of buttermilk.

> *Anxiety and depression.* Many fasters suffer from a kind of emo-
tional hangover. Others are stricken by doubts, worrying that
they have undertaken too much. These feelings can be easily
dispelled by engaging in activities that help you the most in such
situations. You should not force yourself to do anything, but
you should also not let yourself be overwhelmed by your wor-
ries. For safety's sake, during your second day of fasting be sure
to take a wide detour around all grocery stores and restaurants.

The Third Day of Fasting

Starting with the third day of your fast, you will feel stronger,
more secure, and more confident. Even if you are still bothered
by changes here and there, you will overcome them quickly, just
as you did on the second day. After all, with each passing day you
experience more clearly how seamlessly your internal controls are
functioning and how easily your body has adjusted to this new way
of life. Just like anyone else following a normal nutritional regimen, now you can do anything you would like to do.

The third day, at the latest, is time for a cleansing of the intestines by enema, because the intestines usually do not continue to
function on their own; if they do, it is generally at an unsatisfac-
tory level.

WHAT IS PERMITTED?
On page 40 you can review
what you are permitted to
consume during your fast
and what else you should
keep in mind.

The Other Days of Fasting

On the fourth and fifth days of your fast you will feel so well that
you would like more than anything to keep on fasting for another
few days. Do not yield to this urge! For now, stick with this one
week of fasting.

At the very least, schedule another enema to cleanse the
intestines on the fifth day of your fast. Fasters who suffer from
constipation or gastrointestinal problems fast better and with
fewer complaints using daily enemas.

The five fast days are followed by the dietary build-up days,
which are just as important as the fast days and require the same
care and planning as the fasting days did (see pp. 75–85).

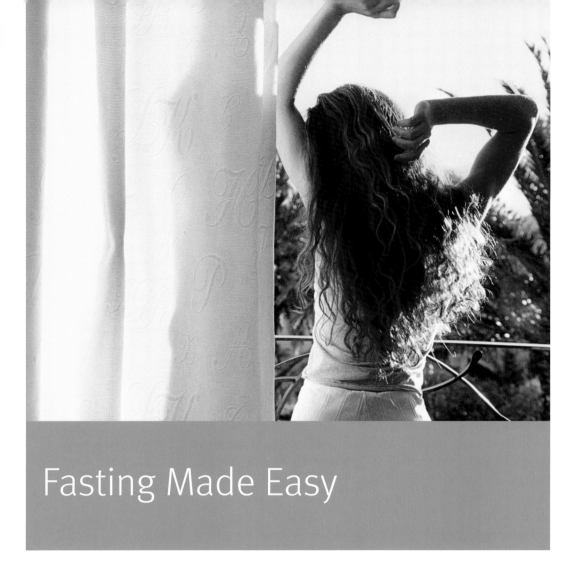

Fasting Made Easy

Fasting means far more than abstaining from food. Fasting is a holistic process. While it is true that the cardiovascular system and muscles of a person who is fasting continue to function normally, often they simply do not react as quickly as they usually do. If, for example, you are a person who jumps right out of bed in the morning when your alarm rings, it is certainly possible that you might become dizzy, and feel faint or ill, with the result that you soon find yourself back in bed.

Begin Your Day with Care

To combat the morning sluggishness brought on by your fast, start the day carefully:

> While still in bed, stretch vigorously, both tightening and releasing your muscles, and yawn heartily.
> Before you get up, first sit on the edge of the bed for a few moments.
> Splash cold water on your face.
> Indulge yourself with a short, peaceful walk in the fresh air. Breathe deeply and regularly through your nose.

If your blood pressure is too low during your fast, or if you would just like to pamper yourself, try the following morning activities.

Following in the Footsteps of Sebastian Kneipp

Sebastian Kneipp was one of the great early pioneers of naturopathy. One of the cornerstones of his teachings on health is that brief exposure to cold stimuli boosts circulation and reinforces the body's own powers of healing. To experience this for yourself, wash your entire body from head to toe with cold water, or take a quick cold shower. Then quickly get into bed without drying yourself off. Alternatively, give yourself a cold arm and face bath following a hot shower; begin at your fingertips, working up to your elbows, and then splash three handfuls of cold water on your face.

Five Minutes of Morning Gymnastics

Light exercise in the morning also stimulates the cardiovascular system. Movements that stretch the muscles, loosen stiff joints, adjust the spine, and at the same time lift your mood are all suitable for this. Music is a good accompaniment.

An Air Bath before an Open Window

Rub your body down with a rough terry-cloth towel, using long vigorous strokes, or with a sturdy bath brush or bristled glove. Begin at the tips of your fingers and toes, and keep rubbing toward

COLD STIMULI
After getting up, walk barefoot in the dew or snow, if the weather permits. Then slip back into bed for 10 minutes and enjoy feeling how your tingling limbs are warming up again.

the heart. Continue doing this for 5 to 10 minutes, after which you will feel comfortably warm. Your cardiovascular system will be stimulated and steady.

Your Body's Own Waste Removal Service

While you are fasting, all the body's "sluices" are open. Emptying the bowels on the first day of your fast by no means completes the process of the body's self-cleansing. Instead, throughout the fast your body will rid itself, through all the openings and pores of the skin, of the metabolic residues and waste products that have been accumulating over the years.

Elimination by the Bowels

The bowel, one of the more important and most sensitive organs, is designed to take in nutrition and eliminate waste. For cleansing and detoxification during a fast, the bowel requires irrigation by enema every other day.

The Self-Administered Enema

An enema might seem old-fashioned, yet it is still the gentlest and most effective method of caring for your bowels. It contributes materially to your well-being while you are fasting and provides quick relief for hunger pangs and headaches or limb pain. Aside from this, the enema continues to be regarded as one of the more important natural home remedies for the entire family in cases of fever and other ailments. Admittedly, an enema is not to everyone's liking, but you will discover that it really is not difficult to administer and that it can bring considerable relief.

In administering an enema, remember these points:

> Fill the enema bag or syringe in the bathroom with 1 quart (1 L) of water at body temperature. Then discharge a test release into the toilet or sink until there are no more air bubbles in the tube.

> Clamp the tube off, either by bending it sharply or by closing the valve (if applicable). Lubricate the rectal tube lightly at the end of the hose (e.g., with Vaseline), and hang the prepared enema bag on a doorknob or towel rack.

IMPORTANT
With the exception of the first day of the fast, do not ingest any Glauber's salt (sodium sulfate), because it would only irritate the bowel anew.

> Position yourself on your hands and knees on the floor and introduce the lubricated rectal tube as deeply as possible into the anus, exerting a little pressure against it.
> Try not to tense up while you let the water flow in slowly. Keep your abdominal wall relaxed and breathe regularly, and then carefully remove the rectal tube when done.
> After two to five minutes, you will feel a strong urge to defecate. The water and the contents of the bowel will be expelled in two to three diarrhea-like streams.

When an Enema Is Not Possible

If you cannot self-administer an enema, other purgative methods are helpful:

> Every morning during your fast, take Epsom salts (2 teaspoons Epsom salts in 1 glass of warm water).
> For people with active bowels, drinking 1 glass (about 4 oz. [1/8 L]) of sauerkraut juice, whey, or buttermilk, as recommended on the first fasting day, can be enough to cleanse the intestines.

SAUNA

If you visit the sauna regularly, you can continue to do so, as long as your cardiovascular system is stable and you limit yourself to two sauna visits of 10 minutes each, with sufficient recovery time in between. After leaving the sauna, use both hands to splash cold water on your face, but not on your legs.

NATURAL ELIMINATION

Find out for yourself which method of elimination you prefer and that seems most helpful.

> Under no circumstances should you take a chemical laxative. Remember that most of the customary laxatives, even salts, can significantly disrupt the quiet work of the intestines.

As long as you are fasting, the intestines will eliminate toxins, and they will continue to do so as long as 20 days afterward.

> Never take diuretics. They upset your well-regulated but sensitive water balance and only give the illusion of helping for one to two days.

Elimination by the Bladder

During a fast, urine can at times take on a dark color and give off a pungent odor. If this is the case, drink clear water to help flush out the kidneys and the urinary tract. For this purpose you need to drink more water than your thirst demands, because urine should be as light in color as possible.

Sometimes you will void a lot of urine, and sometimes only a little, but both are normal. Whether your body retains fluids or passes them can be seen from whether or not you lose weight. Do not become annoyed if your weight remains the same. This can be a sign that your body needs this quantity of fluid for the detoxification processes you have started.

What Is Eliminated through the Skin

As a large surface, the skin has all kinds of work to do during a fast. The less-than-pleasant odors our pores give off only hint at what else is secreted into our undergarments in addition to our sweat. Underwear should therefore be made from absorbent material and able to absorb these effluvia.

When you fast, you will want to wash, shower, and bathe frequently. Bathing is an absolute hygienic necessity before using the sauna or swimming in a pool.

> Your skin will dry out as you fast, so protect it with botanical oils each time after you wash, bathe, or shower.
> Do not use any creams, moisturizing lotions, or makeup with chemical additives during your fast. They block the pores, thereby preventing your skin from breathing and excreting.
> Be conservative with deodorants to avoid skin irritations.

You can look forward to how soft and smooth your skin will be after your fast.

Exhaling Metabolic Residues through the Lungs

Every time you exhale, you expel from your body air laden with gaseous metabolic residues. Let your body breathe with your mouth closed. This is best achieved when hiking or going for a walk out in the open air. In addition, you should air out your house regularly and thoroughly. Throw the window or the balcony door

WELCOME WELLNESS
You should indulge your body during your fast: massages, sun lamps, baths, and Kneipp therapy provide variety without putting any strain on your body.

wide open for five minutes every hour and let the fresh air stream in. At night, turn off the heat and sleep with your window open. This has the added benefit that you also provide your brain and organs with the optimal oxygen "nourishment" they need. (This is highly recommended even when you are not fasting.)

Self-Cleansing Action by the Upper Respiratory Tract

Normally the mucous membranes in the nose, throat, and trachea clean themselves. You can promote this self-cleansing process:

> Fresh morning air stimulates blowing your nose, clearing your throat, and expectorating (spitting). Consequently, in the morning it is good practice to breathe deeply at the open window or take a short morning walk. Splashing two handfuls of cold water on your face has a similar effect.
> Take a break from smoking.

Peppermint lozenges will help you get past that "empty feeling" in your mouth. Take advantage of this opportunity to quit smoking completely. Fasting will help you to do this: after three days a cigarette no longer tastes good.

Elimination through the Mouth

When you are fasting, your tongue may develop a grayish-yellow coating; sometimes it may even become discolored brown to black, depending on what your body is eliminating at that moment. Often the teeth and gums have a coating with an unpleasant smell and a pasty-to-bland taste. This is a result of the tonsils and adenoids getting involved in the elimination process. Ways to fight these effects include the following:

> When you are brushing your teeth, also brush your tongue. Rinse your mouth in between brushings with water more frequently than usual, or suck on a slice of lemon several times a day.
> For bad breath, take 1 teaspoon healing earth powder (loess) mixed with some water (mix according to instructions) two to three times a day. It bonds with noxious substances, rendering them odorless.
> Chewing calamus root and fresh herbs (e.g., chives, dill, or parsley) also helps.

SELF-CLEANSING BY THE VAGINA
The mucous membranes of the vagina are also self-cleansing. This may lead to a temporary increase in vaginal discharge while fasting.

Staying Fit While You Fast

What you can accomplish while fasting depends not so much on the fast itself as on your normal ability to perform. You have this potential as a result of the internal energy supply you can draw on even while you are fasting.

Physical Activity

During a fast you can do almost everything you would normally be able to do. Try it: if you are older, you most likely go for walks; if you are handicapped, you will do whatever you can do; if you are an athlete, you can continue to pursue your usual activities. The best news is that during your fast you can start exercising, even if you did not exercise regularly before. You should, however, be aware of certain minor differences in the use of your physical strength:

> Any activity that requires a quick burst of physical strength—such as running up the stairs, sprinting after a departing train, playing soccer, or skiing—might be difficult during your fast, because these activities are too hard on your cardiovascular system. Recommended instead are the so-called gentle endurance types of sports, such as Nordic walking, running, swimming, hiking, bicycling, rowing, slow-paced mountain climbing, or cross-country skiing.

> No matter which sport you prefer, during your fast you should push yourself at least once every day to the upper limits of your abilities. This ensures that your existing performance level is fully maintained even during your fast.

Can I Enhance My Performance during a Fast?

Your challenged muscles will grow through endurance training, while your body weight drops. Is this a paradox? No, because both strength and performance obey the law of demand or function. What is functioning will not be broken down; in fact, with appropriate demands it can even be built up, because the well-nourished person who is fasting has adequate protein reserves available. What

BREAKING DOWN FAT

After only a few minutes of endurance training, your body burns superfluous fat effectively and builds muscles. Moreover, your head clears, your mood improves, and your breathing flows smoothly. It is more fun with a partner. After your fast, look for kindred spirits at a sports club in your neighborhood or in the classified ads of your daily paper or on an Internet site.

is then broken down to extract energy is only fat and superfluous weight that limits movement. Anyone who remains primarily in bed during a fast will lose strength and fitness, just like someone who eats three meals a day but who does not move. Many people have experienced this process firsthand when they have spent time sick in bed.

Endurance training with the goal of improving performance is just as possible during a fast as at any other time and follows the same rules:

> Train consistently every day.
> Train all muscle groups equally.
> Begin slowly and gradually increase the intensity.
> Push your performance limits once or twice a day, every day.
> Pay attention to the harmonious transitions between phases of stress and phases of rest.

TIP FOR SUCCESS

Obviously, everyone has not only physical but also emotional "baggage," so do not get worried if you experience depressing dreams of war, blood, or filth; nasty thoughts; aggressive moods; melancholy states of mind.

> Most people experience a change in their sleeping habits during a fast. Although their sleep is more relaxed, everything that has been accumulated in their thoughts comes to the surface all the more clearly. This means that you will be much more conscious of your dreams.
> It is important to discuss what is burdening you if this happens. Write it down if you do not have anyone to talk to, then later go back and, in the light of day, look at what you have written. Come to grips with your emotional "baggage." You will see how this examination can unburden you. Keeping a diary has been helpful for many people. When you read it after your fast, you will be amazed at all the unsettling thoughts that have flowed from you.

Here are two examples from medically supervised fasts:

> A 54-year-old man, a 10K runner, trained daily during his 50-day fast. On the 49th day of his fast he ran his personal best time.
> An athletic 40-year-old man fasted 21 days, losing 24 pounds in the process. With daily gymnastics, tennis, swimming, and hours of hiking, he returned home in top condition. The following year he returned for another fast with his leg in a cast due to an accident. This time, as far as athletic activities were concerned, he was virtually unable to do anything but walk with a cane and do some gymnastics in his room. Although the cast was removed at the end of his fast and he had again lost 24 pounds after his 21-day fast, he was weak. He had to learn to walk again, and he regained his previous condition only after six weeks of intense training.

Although the indolent and sluggish can achieve the same weight loss as those who are active, they have broken down not

TIP FOR SUCCESS

By all means, lie down for an afternoon nap. A liver compress will assist the liver in its important detoxification function.

> Fill a hot water bottle flat with hot water and press to remove the remaining air. Now fold a linen towel lengthwise once, dip one third of it into hot water, and wring it out.
> Lie down and spread the moist portion of the towel in the area of your liver. Place the hot water bottle on the towel, and cover it with the dry part of the towel. Cover your entire body well.
> Where you spend your resting time does not matter. What is important, however, is to lie down, rest, relax, and stay warm. Simply lying down increases the blood circulation in your liver by 40 percent.

only fat but also muscle. No wonder their blood pressure is unstable and they feel increasingly lethargic! Nor is it surprising that these people cannot maintain the gains they achieved with fasting, and so they quickly regain weight after their fasts.

Mental and Artistic Performance

Naturally, during a fast you can perform mental activities as well as physical ones. You are absolutely capable of being artistically creative—often with far better results than usual. For example, an 82-year-old comes to mind who experienced an exceptionally intensive creative phase during a fast. And an Austrian philosopher insisted that he wrote his best works while fasting. Several painters even claimed that, during their fasting, they went through especially productive phases, while others experienced revelations of color and form that they later transformed into paintings.

Rest and Relax

By alternating regularly between tension and release, between movement and resting, a state of physical and psychological well-being can be achieved most quickly. For this reason you should rest after every exertion, every bath, and every sauna visit, massage, or other activity. Do not read, watch television, or work at your computer; instead, you should really rest. Close your eyes. Exhale. Rest. Give your body time for its metabolic work of breaking down, transforming, and building up. Your body needs rest to accomplish this. So the rule during a fast is to observe a rest period three times every day.

Letting Go

Anyone who has learned to let go and relax will overcome difficulties more easily. During a fast the body is naturally inclined to relax. For this reason a fast is an ideal time to learn the art of relaxing and concentrating on your own body. Autogenic training, yoga, breathing techniques, and other relaxation methods can help.

TOTALLY RELAXED

Here are just three of the myriad methods for relaxing:

> Yoga relaxes and loosens muscles and also makes you supple. It supports blood circulation, makes your skin attractively rosy, lets breathing flow smoothly again, and at the same time strengthens your muscles.

> The Feldenkrais Method makes you aware of ingrained habits of posture, movement, and thought and also brings the body and mind into their natural balance.

> Autogenic training is one of the more effective means of leaving stress and hectic activity behind. In addition, it has a positive influence on both body and mind.

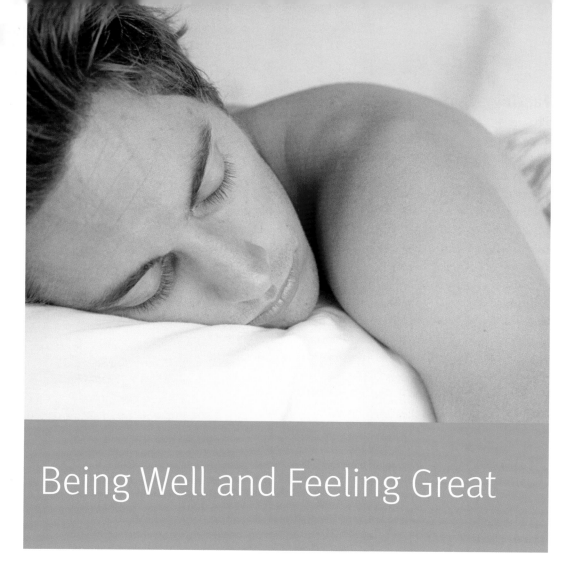

Being Well and Feeling Great

If you fast, you may have difficulty sleeping. Do not complain. Use the time. Fortunately, though, not even half of the people who fast are kept awake at night more often than usual. Most sleep deeply and soundly, even if not as long as they normally do. For many who previously suffered from sleep disorders, their sleeping habits become regularized during their fasts. Many people who fast can noticeably improve their ability to fall asleep or sleep through the night by temporarily abstaining from nourishment.

Fasting Nights

Prepare yourself for the oncoming night by switching off, consciously relaxing, and winding down the day. Avoid stimulating or upsetting activities such as television, Internet, or video games shortly before bedtime. Instead, take a short walk or sit in a comfortable chair to read or listen to music—in short, do something that makes you happy and relaxed. All the images you have taken in will continue to have an effect during your sleep, even if you are not consciously aware of this and cannot remember anything the next day.

Here are a few more ways to promote falling asleep:

> **Unburden your mind**. You can help to drain the increased blood flow to the brain after intellectual work or a lively discussion by taking an evening walk in the fresh air, "water-treading" in the bathtub (cold water, calf-high), taking a footbath that gradually increases in temperature (see p. 57), or doing a few push-ups or squats. Any physical activity redirects the excess blood from the head to the muscles.

> **"Cold feet do not sleep well."** Read how you can remedy this quickly, on page 57.

> **"Closed windows invite nightmares."** Lack of oxygen can lead to bad dreams, so turn off the heat and sleep with the windows wide open. If you become cold, unless it is dangerously cold outside, do not close the window, but put another blanket on your bed.

> **Sleeping pills? Painkillers?** Avoid them as much as you possibly can. If need be, have your accustomed prescription medications ready on your night table. If you are suffering, take one, but before you do that, try to do everything you can to encourage sleep in the natural way.

TIP
The best herbal teas to induce a gentle sleep:
> Lavender
> Hops
> Lemon balm
> St. John's wort
> Valerian

When You Have Trouble Sleeping

Sound and healthy sleep can be seriously impaired by physical discomfort, stomach trouble, and anxiety. As a rule, though, you can help yourself to enjoy peaceful sleep once again. Consider these facts:

> A full stomach not only blocks mental activity; it will not let you sleep well. Even while fasting, you can experience feelings of fullness created by gas and discomfort from cramps, especially during the time immediately following your fast. What helps most is a cold, wet Priessnitz compress (see sidebar).

> If you are tossing and turning, and restlessness forces you to get up, use a washcloth to wipe yourself down from head to toe with cold water; do not take a shower. Then go back to bed without drying yourself. You will be amazed at how well and how quickly this simple remedy works.

> Sleep during a fast can become shallower and shorter. Reread the motto at the beginning of this chapter again: "Do not complain" (p. 54). If you should wake up at a time you are not normally awake, do not become irritated. Accept being awake. Look at this in a positive light: how often do you get time to read, think, or write undisturbed?

The Time Is Not Lost

Use the time. Enjoy the still of the night or the dawning of the day. If thoughts of your family, work, or life come to mind, accept them. Do not resist thinking about yourself. Keep a pen and paper handy, and write down the thoughts that come to mind. Many people have found the path to the self or the keys to long-sought solutions to problems during such nights of fasting. Why not read a little? How often does the pressure of daily life prevent you from having the time? Now you have it. The next morning, you will notice that you are not even tired.

As a general rule, people who are fasting can make do with five or six hours of sleep, especially if they observe the recommended three rest periods per day. Only those who cannot embrace these nightly waking hours and become irritated from lying awake, believing that sleep is necessary at any cost, will wake the next morning feeling sleep-deprived and unrested. For all their effort, they still probably did not sleep any longer.

TIP FOR SUCCESS

If you suffer from flatulence, a cold wet **Priessnitz compress** will bring relief. Dip one third of a linen towel into cold water, wring it out, and fold it so that there are one moist and two dry layers. Lay the cold wet side on the abdomen and spread a dry folded terry-cloth towel over it. (Your waistband will hold everything in place.)

Keep Yourself Nice and Warm

Do not be surprised if you frequently have cold hands and feet during your fast. Although your "inner furnace" can keep producing as much heat from your body's fat deposits as from nourishment, during your fast it turns down this internal furnace as if it were being forced to conserve the body's reserves.

Here are ways to help yourself:

> Your clothing should be light but warm. Your first choice should be natural, warming, and absorbent fabrics like cotton, muslin, and wool. Underwear should be practical and made from materials that breathe. Choose shoes that have cork or leather soles, and wear wool socks. In summer, open sandals or clogs are an ideal option.

> Physical activity creates heat and, as an added benefit, stimulates your cardiovascular system.

> You will perceive hot beverages as more pleasant than cold ones. Drink plenty of tea or warm vegetable broth.

> A hot liver compress (see p. 52) daily at noon or in the evening will warm you up—and also detoxify the liver.

> If only your feet are cold, warm them up with a hot water bottle or a hot footbath. If you feel cold or chilled to the bone, you will need more: an escalating temperature footbath is the best protection against colds (see the following box).

> During bathing or swimming, the fasting body cools off more rapidly than otherwise. Shorten your swimming time a bit, and make sure to warm up completely.

TIP

Do you want a quick bowl of hot soup now and then, but you do not feel like cooking all the time? Prepare the fasting soup in larger quantities, then freeze it in one-meal portions, which defrost quickly when needed.

THE ESCALATING-TEMPERATURE FOOTBATH

Pour lukewarm (not hot!) water into a bucket up to your calves. Place your feet in the bucket, gradually adding hot water so that the feet keep receiving more heat. After 15 to 20 minutes, your entire body will be charged with heat. At the end, briefly rinse or wash your feet with cold water. Dress warmly or go to bed immediately.

The Fasting Blues . . .

After the first two or three days of their week of fasting, most fasters are relieved, unburdened, and, as a result, feel extremely good. They have gained confidence in their fast, and their amazement at how good they feel turns into elation over their journey into new well-being. Naturally, though, not everything is sunshine and roses; they may also encounter little fasting downturns, frequently in the morning or for a few hours during the day. Feelings like "I feel listless," "I am tired," "I feel a little dizzy," or "I am sluggish" can creep in. Frequently, fasters ask themselves, "What should I do? Pull myself together or let myself go?" The answer is both, but in the proper proportion.

Making the effort to undertake physical activity is especially important for those of us who tend toward corpulence or sluggishness. If you are carrying extra weight, you cannot fully enjoy physical activity. Sluggish people are, as a general rule, out of shape. So it is especially important when fasting to pull yourself together to be active, because with weight loss the muscles become flabby. That is why this is precisely the time for you to become active. The lost pounds ensure that becoming active will not be too difficult. You will see: the day will come when impediments and sluggishness are overcome—the day when activity begins to be really enjoyable, gradually becoming a necessity. Until then, though, remember to make the effort.

Low Blood Pressure

Fasting is usually more difficult for people whose blood pressure is too low (less than 100/60 millimeters of mercury) than for others. Weakness, dizziness, and difficulty concentrating often plague them throughout the fast. Their cardiovascular systems need help:

> Pay attention to the points made in the chapter "Fasting Made Easy" (see pp. 44–53).

> If necessary, drink a cup of mild black tea with a teaspoon of honey, both in the morning and after the liver compress at midday. Preferably, drink the tea while still lying down. Ginseng tea

TIP

An enema is helpful when body and spirit go on strike—for example, in the case of hunger pangs or dizziness. If your bowels work "normally," use lukewarm water; if they tend to be sluggish, the water can be a bit cooler.

or mild wormwood tea are another way to gently stimulate the cardiovascular system.

> Physical activity is very important for stabilizing the cardiovascular system, but start slowly.

. . . And Other Challenges

In contrast to minor lows, genuine fasting crises are rare during short fasts. While they can occur during longer fasting treatments of 20 days or more, even then it is rare that healthy people experience a crisis. More frequently these occurrences happen to fasters who are not well.

Fasting crises come out of the blue. The fasting person suddenly feels listless, irritable, or depressed. Old infirmities flare up, and flulike symptoms appear. On a day like this the body has a lot to do for itself. It wants to be pampered. Bed rest, warmth, and an enema will help most people under these circumstances. Drink plenty of water or tea. A glass of buttermilk, sipped slowly, can work wonders. It would be totally misguided to force yourself into exertion or to break off your fast. Ultimately, fasting crises are therapeutic crises. These are the hours and days when stored toxic substances are being removed from the tissues with particular intensity and are coursing through the body. As soon as these substances have been excreted, the crisis will be over.

TIP FOR SUCCESS

It is highly worthwhile to record the course of your fast in detail in a **Fasting Diary**. Every day you should note all the specifics of your diet, your waste removal, and your physical and mental condition, as well as your physical and mental activities. Write down the major and minor complaints that plagued you before you began your week of fasting. Note, as well, which of these still remain after your fast. Take stock of what your week of fasting has brought you.

What Can Be Different When Fasting?

Bear in mind that, compared with your customary daily life, you are living in a kind of "state of emergency" during your fast. Although your body has no problems with this, some of its functions can change during this period. Perhaps you recognize yourself in one or another of the following examples.

When Your Vision Seems to Weaken

Many fasters occasionally think that their visual acuity is failing; for example, the print blurs on the page. This is because the pressure in the eye decreases somewhat during a fast. This is no cause for concern; everything will be back to normal as soon as the week is over. After a fast the ability to see is often even better than before it.

Attention, drivers: concentration and reaction time can also decline during a fast (see the following caution).

Be Patient

If you have already fasted previously, you may be familiar with this phenomenon from your own experience: you read a paragraph once, twice, a third time, and still cannot understand it. The mental capacity to absorb it seems to be blocked. Do not let this bother you; this too will resolve itself in a few days.

A Time-Out for Your Brain

Another thing that can happen to you during a fast is that, more quickly than usual, you forget what has just been said. Important appointments can also slip your mind. Yes, you can even forget your own telephone number! It might also be a struggle for you to find the right word. No surprise here; even your brain needs a vacation once in a while. Lack of concentration and a reduced capacity to absorb are a normal expression of the fact that your brain is shutting down after previous overload, and that is precisely what it should do and should be permitted to do.

HEADACHES
Headaches during a fast are most often the result of serious dehydration. Are you actually drinking enough liquids? Increase the amount of your fluid intake, and relax.

When You Ought to Pull Yourself Together

Whether it be temporary blues or physical sluggishness, it is important for you not to let yourself go but to pull yourself together. Take a 10-minute walk in fresh air. Usually that will get you over your low point. If this listless feeling does not disappear despite walking, physical activity, or games there is still plenty of time to let yourself relax. Then it is appropriate to withdraw to a quiet room, lie down, read, or sleep.

Regarding Sexual Potency

Even sexual stamina can undergo a temporary change through fasting. Whether it is reduced or enhanced varies from person to person. One thing is certain, however: after the fast, your libido will definitely be stronger and balanced, more normal than before.

Irregular Periods

Fasting can postpone a woman's period. If you use natural contraception methods, your usual practice of identifying "conception-free" days is not reliable. If you are sexually active during your fast, be absolutely sure to use additional protection. Bleeding itself may be more or less than usual. This, like sexual desire, differs from woman to woman, but here too it is more likely to be normalized after a fast.

HEARTBURN

If fruit juice causes you heartburn, boil 1 tablespoon of flaxseed in 1 pint (0.5 L) of water. After 5 minutes, skim off the froth that has developed and mix it into the juice.

FASTING AND THE YO-YO EFFECT

If at the end of your fast you adhere to the rules for breaking the fast, if you treat your body carefully during the dietary build-up phase, and if you subsequently follow a balanced diet, you do not have to worry about the "yo-yo effect." Only those who fall back into old eating habits after the fast and dietary build-up period will start gaining weight again—and much faster than they would like. Accordingly, allocate enough time to teach yourself about healthy nutrition.

WEIGHT LOSS DURING THE WEEK OF FASTING

Woman:
40 years old
5 ft. 3 in. (1.60 m) tall
Weight at the beginning
of the fast: 143 lb. (65 kg)

Man:
40 years old
5 ft. 9 in. (1.75 m) tall
Weight at the beginning
of the fast: 176 lb. (80 kg)

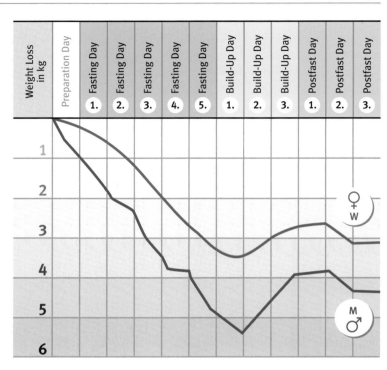

Weight Loss: A Welcome Side Effect

If you decide to fast, you usually want not only to detoxify the body but also to lose a few extra pounds. Consider this example: a man and a woman are fasting because they are moderately overweight. The woman's weight curve shows a regular downward and upward movement. The man's curve, however, drops on the first and third fasting days and then ticks upward more steeply than the woman's on the second and third days of food build-up (see graph). This is typical for people with elevated salt and water content in their tissues. On the fourth fasting day the man's weight loss is virtually zero. His body is retaining water. This, too, is completely normal. Salt deposits in the tissues are dissolved and often excreted by the kidneys only on the following day. In your case, weight can remain unchanged for days, but that is no reason to become discouraged.

You will see the real weight loss resulting from the week of fasting on the morning of the first day after the fast. The woman in our example lost 6.6 pounds (3 kg), and the man 8.8 pounds (4 kg). The woman lost about 4 pounds (1.8 kg) of fatty tissue, whereas the man lost approximately 5.5 pounds of such tissue (2.5 kg). Because 2.2 pounds (1 kg) of fatty tissue yields 6,000 calories, we can calculate that each day the woman had 1,500 calories and the man 2,100 calories available from burning stored fat. This amount is fully adequate to live well, work, play sports, and think. Thus there is no loss of energy, liveliness, or pleasure, despite the weight loss. (One small consolation for women: although men typically lose more weight, they put it back on faster!) Even someone who loses only a small amount of weight enjoys the full benefits of fasting.

Taking Stock of Your Weight

To gain a better overview, record your personal weight history. On the next page you will find Your Personal Weight Chart and Your Personal Weight Curve. This is where you should record your starting weight on the morning of Preparation Day. Weigh yourself every morning during your fast, and enter your weight here. Set strict weighing rules: for example, weigh yourself every morning in your nightgown or pajamas after urinating, or every morning naked after your bowel movement and shower. Whichever method you choose, always maintain the same parameters. Only by doing this can you get an accurate weight assessment, and you will find the final balance on the morning of the first day after your fast.

And If You Have Weight Problems?

Continue to monitor your weight in the weeks and months that follow. "Living with the scale" is your surest means for controlling and maintaining your weight. Place the scale at a spot in your bathroom where you cannot miss it. Keep your weight chart and pencil close at hand. Soon, weighing yourself will become a personal ritual.

WHAT YOU GAIN FROM FASTING
Fasting can help you to achieve a greater sense of well-being through reduced fluid retention, reduced salt, detoxification, and a purge of waste products. It also results in improved performance through eliminating excess weight.

Your Personal Weight Chart

Data	Morning of Preparation Day	Weight in Pounds
_____	Morning of 1st Fasting Day	_____
_____	Morning of 2nd Fasting Day	_____
_____	Morning of 3rd Fasting Day	_____
_____	Morning of 4th Fasting Day	_____
_____	Morning of 5th Fasting Day	_____
_____	Morning of 1st Build-Up Day	_____
_____	Morning of 2nd Build-Up Day	_____
_____	Morning of 3rd Build-Up Day	_____
_____	Morning of 1st Postfast Day	_____
_____	After 4 Weeks	_____
_____	After 8 Weeks	_____

Your Personal Weight Curve

Weight Loss (in Lbs.)	1st Fasting Day	2nd Fasting Day	3rd Fasting Day	4th Fasting Day	5th Fasting Day	1st Build-Up Day	2nd Build-Up Day	3rd Build-Up Day	1st Postfast Day	2nd Postfast Day	3rd Postfast Day	4th Week	8th Week
1													
2													
3													
4													
5													
6													
7													
8													

Weight before starting fast _____ lb.
Minus weight on the morning of 1st Postfast Day _____ lb.
Weight lost during the fast _____ lb.

The Brilliance of Detox

This may sound strange at first, but to summarize what was said in the previous chapters, the fasting organism extracts energy and warmth from fat (the body's energy reserve) and draws building materials from the body's own protein. The body does not randomly burn just *any* fat or just *any* protein-containing substance, however. The body breaks substances down in the following order:

> Things that stress it
> Things it does not need
> Things that bother it
> Things that make it ill

Capillary biology research shows that we become ill not only from the long-term excessive consumption of fats and carbohydrates but also from the excessive intake of protein. Excess protein is deposited on the interior walls of the smallest blood vessels, the capillaries, which are found in all organs. On the basis of these deposits (accumulations of toxins) it is now possible to see the often still-unnoticed precursors to many diseases that years from now can lead to cardiovascular impairment and, at worst, to a heart attack or stroke.

Similar deposits are found in the connective tissue, that is, the cushioning between all organs, muscles, and joints. The consequences are painful diseases such as the commonest forms of rheumatoid arthritis and nonarticular rheumatism, to name two examples.

WHAT THE BODY WILL NEVER METABOLIZE
The body will never metabolize:
> What is needed—such as the heart or muscle system.
> What is functioning—such as all activities of the organs
> What is essential for life—such as the body's control mechanisms

The real secret of fasting is hidden behind this natural law, which is programmed into the human body. We can safely depend on our own bodies' internal reliability.

Fasting for Preventive Purposes

We can do something to fight these dangers by getting our bodies to break down unneeded protein from time to time. This is what happens when we fast. At the same time, we must also learn not to overload our protein reserves again immediately after the fast. Thus fasting and a customized meal plan are integral parts of the same regimen.

The Process of Detoxification

Detoxification is also linked to the same metabolic processes as the breaking down of substances. Toxins are bonded to fat and protein and are deposited in the connective tissue. This bond is broken through the metabolism of fat and protein during a fast. The toxins then can be excreted through the bowels, kidneys, and skin.

Now you can understand why it is misguided to enrich fasting beverages with protein or to consume "protein drinks." Doing this would hinder the waste removal process and deprive us of a chance for healing. Protein supplements for extremely overweight people during long fasts (longer than 30 days—these should be done only at a fasting clinic) are a different matter entirely. Such cases are predominantly concerned with weight loss and less about waste removal and detoxification. A protein supplement is also certainly a sensible choice for older people.

Assessing the Overall Benefits

In addition to the factors already mentioned, weight loss through fasting can lead to a variety of changes in the body. For example, it reduces the strain on the knee joints, feet, and spinal discs—in short, the weight-bearing elements of the body. It takes stress off the heart, which can now pump better and more powerfully. Breathing becomes freer. The lungs can take in more oxygen, and the cardiovascular system can deliver it faster to all the tissues. High blood pressure returns to normal. Although blood pressure that is too low can temporarily cause some fatigue or dizziness, it soon stabilizes at an appropriate level. During the first five days of a fast, temporarily elevated blood sugar decreases to normal but never goes below that. An excessively high level of blood lipids (e.g., cholesterol, triglycerides, and other substances) declines with each day of fasting. As soon as blood lipid values are normal, deposited fat is removed from the liver cells and the blood vessels and from all the fatty organs. Thus removal of fat occurs not only "externally" but also "internally" (therapeutic fasting begins with this; see pp. 103–111). Even when laboratory tests have shown

IMPORTANT
Diabetic persons requiring medication and people suffering from liver disease should go to a fasting clinic. They should not fast independently.

slightly elevated liver values, you can be sure that they will have improved after five days of fasting, though only if you have totally given up alcohol, which should be regarded as completely taboo during a fast anyway. In short, it can be said that the normalizing tendency of the body's self-correction is reflected by normalized laboratory and test data.

If you gradually trim excess weight down to an almost normal weight and at the same time make sure to get sufficient physical activity, you have done a great deal for your own health. With every pound lost, the cited risk factors are reduced. With every day of fasting, your body is detoxified. The result: healthy and valuable years have been added to your life span (see also pp. 98–101).

TIP FOR SUCCESS

Blood uric acid levels (purine) increase during a fast, a sign that a particularly intense cell breakdown and alteration is now under way. Only five to six days after the fast ends, the uric acid level in the blood will decrease again.

A small number of people cannot handle these elevated levels very well. If you have been aware of elevated uric acid levels in your blood for a while, you should very strictly observe a few rules during your fast:
> Drink plenty of fluids and eat two to three lemons a day, either squeezed as juice or in slices to suck on from time to time. Although acidic in raw form, lemon juice counteracts hyperacidity when the body metabolizes it. That puts lemons, like most fruit, in the alkaline category of foods.
> Steer clear of alcoholic beverages. They are harmful during any fast.
> Evacuate your bowels especially well.
> If your physician has placed you on preventative antigout, uric-acid reducing medication, you must continue to take it during the fast. Accordingly, you should not fast independently in this case, but instead go to a fasting clinic.

Cosmetics from the Inside Out

A fasting doctor always finds it impressive to see how the face of a fasting person changes. After only five days of fasting, the puffy "full-moon face" with feverish red blotches begins to relax and regain its characteristic contours. Dull eyes become clear; restless glances become steady. A growing self-confidence can be read in the features. During a fast the fatigued, resigned, gray face of the person suffering from exhaustion first turns inward, becomes quiet, and collapses a bit. Then, though, it fills out, gaining a freshness and delicacy. The eyes begin to sparkle. After this restructuring process the soft, smooth, elastic skin is conspicuous, blemishes have disappeared, and wrinkles are smoothed.

Help for Cellulite

In the course of a lifetime the elastic fibers of the epidermis and hypodermis decrease, as does the elasticity of the supporting and connective tissue. The collagen fibers become thicker and immobile because water, salts, and the body's own waste are trapped between them. When pushed together, tissue that is clogged and laden with toxins in this way results in "orange-peel skin" or cellulite, which is rather painful when it is pinched.

Detoxifying fasting, physical activity, vigorous brushing to stimulate increased blood circulation, and oiling the skin after alternating hot and cold showers can help this condition far more profoundly than superficial cosmetic techniques. These deeper measures can rejuvenate the skin and underlying connective tissues quickly, making them pain-free and tighter.

The same process also takes place inside the body. People losing weight are generally afraid that their skin will become loose and wrinkled. At most this occurs during the fast, but fortunately, after the build-up of food the skin and internal organs tighten up again. After a longer fast many people report that they feel five years younger and their detoxified body is noticeably tighter.

TIP

A massage with natural oils likewise has a detoxifying effect and, if performed regularly, will reduce cellulite. Suitable oils include aloe vera oil, macadamia nut oil, and jojoba oil. Rub a bit of oil between your hands, then with your fingertips lift one area of the skin at a time, compress it slightly, and finally pull it upward until the skin becomes slightly rosy.

How Your Partner Can Help

No matter whether both partners fast together or only one of them chooses to abstain from food, their behavior requires one basic insight: fasting means reaching deep down into yourself, obeying your body's own daily rhythm, and behaving in the way your body requires at the moment, not how your partner may want or expect. When you fast, you can break old habits. You are living by different rules than usual. Give each other space; you will find each other again even more clearly.

> Learn about fasting together. Read this fasting guide together. Discuss the subject in detail.
> Decide together on the time to begin your fast.
> Agree on where you will spend your fast, where you will take your meals, and how you will arrange both your mutual and your personal leisure time, as well as your individual rest periods.
> Change your sleeping habits. During the fast you should sleep in separate rooms, both because of the odors that can arise during fasting and because of possibly different requirements for fresh air. Moreover, with separate rooms you can turn on the light if you cannot sleep, making it possible to read or do something else without disturbing your partner.
> Sexual activity does not have to change during a fast, but it may. Accept the changes in your partner's behavior.
> Respect your partner's desire for rest under all circumstances.
> Personal hygiene requires special attention as a result of changes in body odor.
> Mood swings during a fast are quite normal. Accept these mood swings in your partner, and do not complain if he or she withdraws more frequently than usual.
> Promise your partner to do everything you can to help resist the temptations of food, smoking, or alcohol, and live up to this agreement.

FASTING IN THE WORKPLACE

> When you fast, allow more time than usual during your morning routine to get ready and exercise; if necessary, get up earlier.
> Plan more time for your morning commute; do not rush. Leave your car at home, and if there is public transportation, take the train, bus, or subway. Get off one stop earlier and walk the rest of the way. Use the stairs instead of the elevator. Physical activity and lots of fresh air are important. Also, use your lunch hour for a brisk walk in the fresh air or for a short nap at your desk.

> Keep in mind the changes in your breath and body odor. Rinse your mouth frequently with clear water, chew parsley, suck on a lemon wedge, or eat a (sugarless) peppermint drop.
> At the end of the workday, consciously plunge yourself into your own personal domain and do everything that others do during vacation. Decline visits from curious friends; turn down invitations; go to bed early.
> Get together regularly with other fasters, or exchange your fasting experiences by telephone or e-mail.

Temptations Resisted

We would not be human if our fasting time were not full of temptations: "just a tiny bite," or "one apple really can't hurt." True, the apple cannot do serious harm, yet every little bite, whatever it is, will jeopardize your fast because it will create a hunger for more. If you provoke your digestive juices, you should not be surprised when they demand something to digest. Consistently not eating really *is* easier; experienced fasters know this.

What about that cup of coffee, which has no calories at all, or an ice cream, which, though it has a lot of calories, does not need to be chewed? The OK cannot be given here either. Coffee, like ice cream, is a strong stimulant for the gastric juices in the stomach; it promotes the production of digestive juices, triggering an appetite just like any other food.

It is truly dangerous for you to succumb to the temptation to eat a full meal with soup, entree, and dessert. A relapse like this can have very serious consequences, ranging from abdominal cramps to cardiovascular collapse (see pp. 90–91). The guidelines for the build-up of food are even more relevant during the fast.

Inner Freedom

Every temptation you conquer makes you strong. The fears and temptations you overcome are precisely what make you mature and grow internally.

Fasting means doing without. You can practice this during your fast. You will find that the ability to do without is ultimately a benefit. Although it is better not to go into town and stand in front of butcher shops and bakeries during the first days of a fast, later you will be able to do so with an amazing inner freedom. You will be able to sit in a restaurant and order a peppermint tea or a glass of hot water and lemon without sugar, or perhaps a glass of freshly squeezed orange juice, and watch others eat without feeling any hunger pangs of your own. Proud as a peacock, you can then return home, strengthened by a well-earned sense of accomplishment.

DAILY RITUALS
Continue to take a break for afternoon tea even after your fast is over. With each sip, try to re-create the feelings of peace, relaxation, and inner freedom you experienced during your week of fasting. Draw strength from this for the rest of the day.

CHANGING YOUR HABITS
Taking a break from smoking and alcohol during your fast is necessary not only for your health but also because it defines this vital question: "Are you the master of your life, or are you a slave to your habits?" Here, too, the same principle applies—a clear and uncompromising "no" at the beginning of your fast makes doing without much easier during your entire fast. Having to say "no" each separate time only torments you unnecessarily later on. At the end of the fast you will have gained so much determination that you will be able to make completely different decisions. Why not simply continue to do without those bad habits? After all, you will have acquired one of humankind's finest abilities: being able to obtain pleasure from very little.

FASTING AS A BUILDING BLOCK FOR LIFE

For many people the resolution to "fast once a year" becomes a strict rule and thus an extremely important aspect of lifetime health. Others embrace fasting for religious reasons; they experience physical cleansing together with purification of the soul, deepened spiritual illumination, and intellectual enhancement. Incorporate fasting in some form into your life; it is good to do, and it simplifies everything to have one guiding principle and then follow it.

Continue Your Fast or Not?

Remember, this book is intended for healthy people. If you have any doubt about your ability to continue fasting, discuss these questions with a physician who has experience with fasting, or with a fasting coach whom you trust. Those who are fasting for the first time should *under no circumstances* exceed the five fasting days and two dietary build-up days discussed here. If this first fast is a positive and wholesome experience for you, then next time you can fast for seven days with three dietary build-up days. Fasting for healthy people ends at 10 days with 6 dietary build-up days (repeat each dietary build-up day). In the case of longer fasts, risks arise that neither you alone nor a doctor not present with you during the fast can assess.

Listen to your inner voice. Go ahead and fast as long as you feel well, believe your fasting is beneficial, and still have "weight reserves"—that is, as long as all the preconditions for an independent fast are met. An important indication of your ability to continue to fast is that your accustomed capacity to perform continues at the same level or, better still, improves. Listen to your body.

Ending an Extended Fast

The longer you fast, the more time you need to reintroduce food. In the case of fasts lasting 5 to 7 days, plan for 3 full days; for 10-day fasts, allow at least 4 to 5 days to build up to normal food consumption. The rule of thumb is that the more carefully you enter into the phase of dietary build-up, the greater the success of your fast.

DOES YOUR BODY NEED ADDITIONAL SUPPLEMENTS?

Your body does not need additional supplements if you have had good nutritional habits prior to your fast. If, however, this is not the case and you are fasting for a longer period (10 days), you should take a high-quality multivitamin, in addition to 1 teaspoon of a mineral salts mixture, both three times a day.

"The longer the better" is the rule for an extended period of food reintroduction; still, in addition to this general guideline a few important nutritional rules should be followed:

> Eat small quantities.
> Eat simply.
> Eat a healthy diet.
> Do not eat anything difficult to digest: no meat yet (perhaps some fish), no sausage or deli meats, no hard cheeses, and nothing baked.

Fasting Facilitates Healthful Eating

Learning to eat correctly is often more important than the fasting itself. Those who fall back into old eating habits should not be surprised at the "yo-yo effect" shown by the weight curve. Perhaps it would be better for you to fast for short periods three times a year and then subsequently practice disciplined moderate eating habits. In this way you can lose weight gradually and maintain your weight better.

How Often Can You Fast?

Provided that you maintain a healthy diet (see pp. 94–97) and are a healthy faster with weight reserves, you can fast every other month. One week fasting, seven weeks eating—why not? The body will grow accustomed to this rhythm. It is a good rule to schedule a week of fasting once or twice a year. Important here, however, is that every build-up of food should give you new incentives for healthy dietary changes. Do not fast without taking another step toward a whole-food diet. So many people today overeat but are undernourished; multiple fasts by themselves would just manipulate them further into these very deficiencies. So fasting should be undertaken only in conjunction with correct eating habits after the fast, which is at least as important as your fasting time.

RULES OF THUMB FOR THE POSTFAST PERIOD

> Morning: Bircher muesli or uncooked cracked wheat cereal (for recipes, see pp. 81 and 84)
> Noon: Raw fruits or vegetables before the meal
> Evening: Eat lightly and not too late.
> At all times: Rethink your old eating habits.

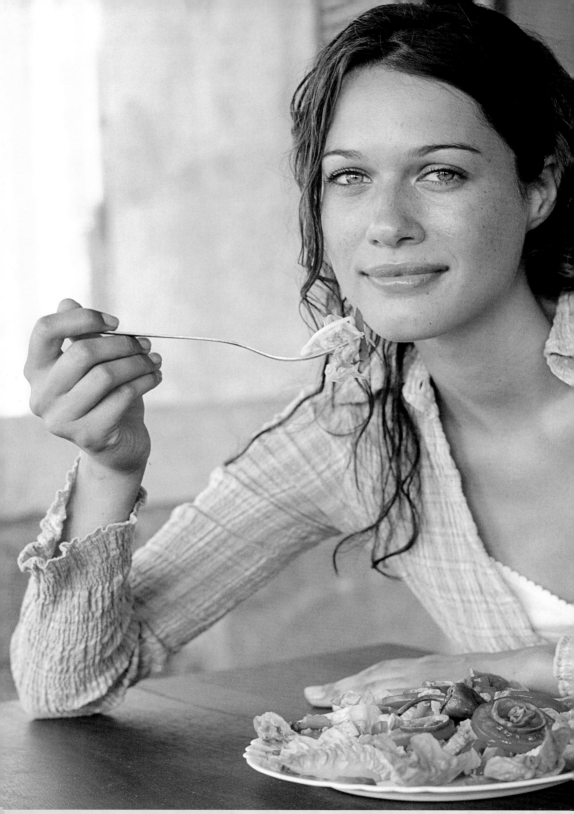

BUILDING UP YOUR DIET

The dietary build-up is an integral part of the fasting period. Eat small quantities of foods with the highest nutritional value possible, and do it with pleasure. You will be amazed at how quickly you feel full and satisfied.

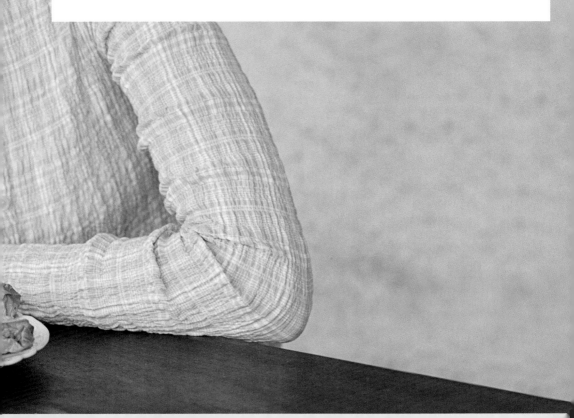

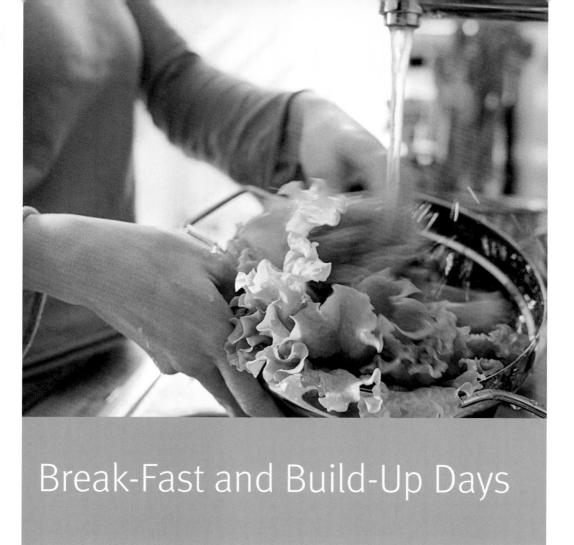

Break-Fast and Build-Up Days

Switching from drinking to eating. George Bernard Shaw, a writer with fasting experience, is said to have claimed that any fool can fast, but only the wise man knows how to break a fast. Why is it so complicated? After all, *build-up* simply means building up your diet and thus reestablishing the everyday metabolic and digestive processes. Yet the switch from eating to fasting is normally quicker than the subsequent switch from fasting to eating.

During the fasting week, your body stopped producing gastric juices. Now it must restart production, which happens gradually, not immediately. Consequently, building up your diet requires as much attention, time, and thoughtfulness as fasting does. To get your digestive juices flowing again and to prevent any problems, you should memorize three fundamental rules for eating: eat slowly, chew well, and eat in silence (see box, p. 78).

At the same time, the dietary build-up days give you an opportunity to reflect on your former eating and drinking habits. Fasting interrupted these habits, and now you may (and can) discard those bad habits you have come to find undesirable. So make some changes: in addition to the fundamental insights you have gained from fasting (i.e., "I feel good and am able to perform well even without eating"), you have now achieved other, new insights during the dietary build-up period. For example, "I need much less food than I did before," or "I don't need as much salt—I can use vegetable seasonings instead." When eating, try to develop new habits based on these experiences.

Your Shopping List

The time has come: your fast is finally drawing to a close. This is why you go food shopping on the fifth fast day. You will be surprised how much pleasure you can get from dealing with food—knowing that you can choose to use it or not, whichever you prefer.

For the three dietary build-up days you will need the following food (per person):

> 1 lb. (500 g) ripe apples, pesticide-free or organic if possible
> 1 head of leaf lettuce
> 8 oz. (250 g) carrots
> 8 oz. (250 g) tomatoes
> 8 oz. (250 g) potatoes

You will also need the corresponding seasonings for recipes starting on page 79. For those who do not like to cook, get one packet each of potato, tomato, or asparagus soup from a health food store or the organic section of your local supermarket.

> 1/2 cup of butter (113.5 g)
> 8 oz. (225 g) flaxseeds

TIP
Food for the eyes—attractive presentation of your food is always important. Avoid using plates that are too large. Using a smaller plate helps to prevent the perception that you do not have enough to eat.

> 1 cup cream cheese (8 oz. [225 g])
> 1 cup (8 oz. [225 g]) low-fat farmer's cheese or cottage cheese
> 2 containers yogurt or organic yogurt (5 oz. [150 g] each)
> 8 oz. (225 g) prunes or figs
> 1 package flatbread, or whole-grain or flaxseed bread
> 1 bottle whey or sauerkraut juice (approximately 1 pint [0.5 L])

If you can find all the fruits and vegetables at a certified organic produce supplier your meals will be much tastier, because fasting fine-tunes your palate. You will also be eating healthier food. If you must eat in a restaurant or cafeteria, choose a dish from the menu that comes closest to the recommendations on the food dietary build-up plan.

Your Meal Plan

The following few pages tell you what you may eat during your next three dietary build-up days. At first it might seem that you are allowed very little food, but you will be amazed how full you will feel from it. Also, during the build-up phase, you should be drinking plenty of fluids, and naturally only those tried and true beverages such as unsweetened teas, water, and diluted fruit juices.

First Build-Up Day

Morning: Morning tea (herbal tea or weak black tea)

Late morning: 1 ripe apple (maybe even sautéed) to break your fast

Noon: 1 bowl potato vegetable soup (see p. 79 for recipe)

Afternoon: Beverage (fruit tea)

Evening: Tomato soup (see p. 80 for recipe), buttermilk with 1 teaspoon flaxseed, 1 slice flatbread

---

IMPORTANT
All recipes for the dietary build-up days are calculated for one portion.

TIP FOR SUCCESS

Focus your entire attention on nutrition. Practice this at every meal, as if you were going to be tested on your ability to eat right.

Take your time. Ignore the clock. Eat in peace—eating is now the most important factor determining your daily schedule.

Chew thoroughly. Digestion begins in the mouth. Chew each piece of solid food 35 times until it liquefies. Gulping your food is bad for you.

Eat in silence. This is the only way you can enjoy your food and leave the table feeling full and satisfied.

Potato Vegetable Soup

1 small potato (about 2 oz. [60 g]) | 1 piece each (1 oz. [30 g])
carrot, leek, and celery root | 1 pinch each freshly ground nutmeg
and marjoram | 1/2 teaspoon yeast flakes | granulated vegetable
bouillon | 1 teaspoon chopped parsley

1 Scrub, peel, and rinse the potato and vegetables, and cut into
thin slices.
2 In a saucepan, bring 1 cup (8 oz. [0.25 L]) water to a boil. Cook
the vegetables covered for 15 minutes until soft.
3 Season the soup to taste with spices, yeast flakes, and granulated bouillon (if needed). Sprinkle with parsley.

Unlike during your fast, it is
no longer necessary to purée
the soups, as you can once
more enjoy solid food during
build-up days.

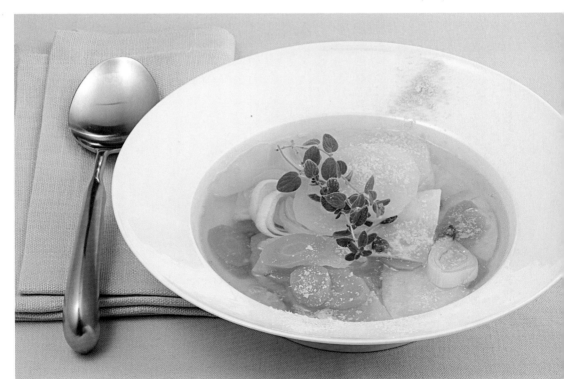

**PREPARE FOR
TOMORROW**
Soften two prunes or
one fig in ½ cup (0.5 L)
water, cover, and let stand
overnight.

Tomato Soup

8 oz. (250 g) ripe tomatoes | 1/2 onion | 1 teaspoon oil |
granulated vegetable bouillon | 1 pinch each sea salt, freshly
ground white pepper, and dried thyme | 1/2 teaspoon yeast flakes
| 1 teaspoon tomato paste | 1 teaspoon chopped parsley, chives,
or thyme

1 Wash and dice the tomatoes, cutting out the stem bases. Peel
the onion and dice finely.
2 Heat the oil, add the diced onion and tomatoes, and sauté for
about 10 minutes until soft. Press the contents through a sieve.
3 In the meantime, bring 1 cup (8 oz. [0.25 L]) water to a boil.
Sprinkle with the granulated bouillon to taste and add the puréed
tomato mixture. Flavor with spices, yeast flakes, and tomato paste,
and then garnish with the fresh herbs.

Energy from the sun: fresh
tomato soup tastes like summer
and warms you up!

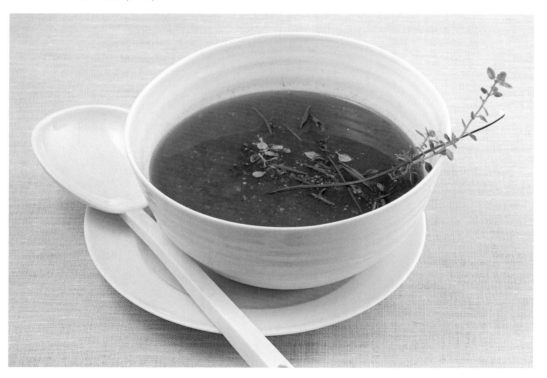

Second Build-Up Day

Morning: 1 glass sauerkraut juice or whey, softened dried fruit from the night before, cracked wheat soup

If you are really hungry: 2 oz. (50 g) yogurt cheese with herbs and 2 slices of flatbread

Late morning: Plenty of fluids (mineral water)

Noon: Leaf lettuce, boiled potatoes, carrots, organic yogurt with sea buckthorn and flaxseeds

Afternoon: Plenty of fluids

Evening: Raw carrots, grain and vegetable soup, sour milk with flaxseeds, 1 slice flatbread

The recipes for these dishes can be found on the following pages.

Cracked Wheat Cereal

2 teaspoons fine cracked wheat | 1 pinch sea salt | 1 tablespoon freshly chopped mixed herbs (e.g., parsley, chives)

1 Heat the cracked wheat in a saucepan over a low flame without browning it. Add 1 cup (8 oz. [0.25 L]) water and bring to a boil. Turn down flame immediately and let wheat simmer, covered, at low heat for about 10 minutes to absorb the liquid. If any liquid remains in the pot, place the cracked wheat in a sieve and let it drain.
2 Enhance the flavor by seasoning the cereal with salt and herbs to taste.

Leaf Lettuce

1/4 head leaf lettuce | 1 pinch each sea salt and freshly ground white pepper | 1/2 teaspoon fruit vinegar or lemon juice | 1 teaspoon sunflower oil | 1 teaspoon chopped chives

1 Pull lettuce leaves apart; clean and rinse the individual leaves carefully under running water. Let the lettuce drain thoroughly in a sieve or spin it in a salad spinner and put it in a bowl.
2 Make a dressing from the salt, pepper, vinegar or lemon juice, and oil. Drizzle onto the salad and toss well. Sprinkle the chopped chives on top.

TIP
If you prefer that your cracked wheat cereal be sweet, add the softened prune or fig cut into small pieces.

Boiled Potatoes

3 small potatoes | caraway seeds

1 Scrub the potatoes thoroughly under running water with a vegetable brush.

2 Bring a sufficient amount of water to a boil in a small saucepan. Add the caraway and boil or steam the potatoes for 20 to 25 minutes until they are done. (If you are preparing the potatoes in a pot with a steamer basket, put the caraway into the steamer water.)

3 Peel the potatoes while they are still hot.

Cooked Carrots

4 oz. (100 g) carrots | 3 teaspoons vegetable broth or water | 1 pinch each sea salt and freshly ground nutmeg | 1 teaspoon sunflower oil | 1 teaspoon freshly chopped parsley

1 Scrub the carrots thoroughly under running water with a vegetable brush, peel if desired, and cut into thin slices.

2 Bring the vegetable broth or water to a boil and cook the carrot slices in it for about 10 minutes until soft.

This constitutes your first solid meal: leaf lettuce as an "appetizer" followed by cooked carrots and boiled potatoes.

3 Remove from heat and season the carrots lightly with salt and nutmeg.

4 Stir in the sunflower oil and sprinkle the carrots with the chopped parsley.

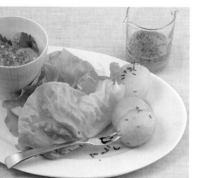

Organic Yogurt with Sea Buckthorn and Flaxseeds

1 cup organic yogurt (1.5 percent low-fat) | 1 teaspoon sea buckthorn juice sweetened with honey | 1 heaping teaspoon flaxseeds

1 Put the organic yogurt and the sweetened sea buckthorn juice into a dessert dish and mix well. If desired, place in the refrigerator until ready to serve.

2 Sprinkle the flaxseeds on the sea buckthorn yogurt just before serving.

Raw Carrots

2 tablespoons sour cream | 1–2 teaspoons lemon juice | several lemon balm leaves | 4 oz. (100 g) carrots | 1/2 apple | 1 lettuce leaf

1 Wash the lemon balm, pat dry, and chop. Then stir chopped lemon balm and lemon juice thoroughly into the sour cream.
2 Scrub the carrots thoroughly under running water with a vegetable brush, peel if desired, and grate them into the sauce using a fine vegetable grater.
3 Wash the apple, cut into quarters, and remove the core. Grate quarters into the sauce.
4 Mix all ingredients and serve on the washed lettuce leaf.

Grain and Vegetable Soup

1/2 small onion | 1 teaspoon olive oil | 1 tablespoon fine cracked wheat | 1 cup (8 oz. [0.25 L]) vegetable broth or water | 2 oz. (50 g) celery root (celeriac) | 1 pinch each sea salt and dried lovage | 1 teaspoon freshly chopped parsley

1 Peel the onion and chop into small pieces.
2 Heat the oil in a pot and fry the onion in it. Add cracked wheat and brown slightly. Cool down by adding the broth or water. Bring everything to a brief boil and let the cracked wheat absorb the liquid over low heat for about 10 minutes.
3 Wash, peel, and finely grate the celery root. Season the cracked wheat soup with salt and lovage. Garnish with celery root and parsley.

Sour Milk (Clabber) with Flaxseeds

3 tablespoons sour milk | 1 teaspoon sea buckthorn sweetened with honey | 1 heaping teaspoon flaxseeds | 1 slice flatbread

Stir sour milk with sea buckthorn juice until smooth and pour into a small bowl. Sprinkle with flaxseeds shortly before serving. Eat with flatbread.

After fasting, your sense of taste is so sensitive that the sour milk with flaxseeds hardly needs to be sweetened.

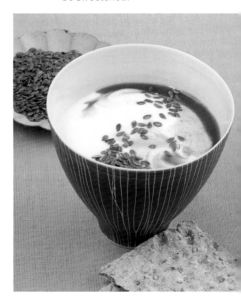

Third Build-Up Day

From your third dietary build-up day on, you are back on the path to good nutrition. There is no better time than right after a fast for correcting your former dietary mistakes.

First, decide what you need and want as far as food is concerned. Would you prefer a fresh salad, or would you rather have hot food? Below are three recommendations.

Recommendation 1: Fresh Raw Food

This option works for anyone who likes raw food and wants to continue to lose weight over the long term (the intake is approximately 800 calories per day). Important: fresh raw food must be prepared fresh, eaten fresh, and chewed thoroughly.

Morning: Morning tea; later, Bircher muesli (soften freshly cracked grain the evening before; see recipe below)

Late morning: Plenty of fluids (if you are hungry, eat as much fresh fruit as you wish)

Noon: Large fresh vegetable platter (leaf lettuce and beets with horseradish) and 1 boiled potato

Afternoon: Plenty of fluids (if you are hungry, eat 1 apple and 12 hazelnuts [filberts] or walnuts)

Evening: Large fresh fruit and/or vegetable platter, containing what you like to eat

Beginning today, start your day with a spring in your step, eating freshly prepared Bircher muesli.

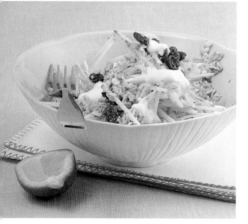

Bircher Muesli: For Fresh Produce Day

1/2 cup milk or yogurt | 1 small apple | 2 teaspoons thick rolled oats | 1 teaspoon grated nuts | 1 teaspoon honey or soaked raisins | 1 teaspoon lemon juice

1 Pour milk or yogurt into a small bowl.
2 Wash and dry the apple; cut in half and remove the core. Grate it unpeeled or cut into small pieces.
3 Mix the apple, rolled oats, and nuts into milk or yogurt; stir well.
4 Add the honey (or the drained raisins) and flavor with lemon juice.

Recommendation 2: A Meal in a Flash

This variation (consisting of approximately 1,000 calories per day) is particularly well suited to people with jobs, to students, and to "fast-food cooks" who have limited time for preparing food and do not want to spend a lot of time in the kitchen.

On an empty stomach: satisfy your thirst; drink water.

Morning: 2 softened prunes or 1 fig, cracked wheat cereal with a dash of milk (see p. 81). Start preparations for lunch: place coarsely cracked spelt (look for spelt in health food stores) in the soup pot you just used on the still-warm stove, and bring to a boil. Keep the pot slightly warm or, as was done in earlier days, wrap it in a blanket and place it in bed or on an armchair so that the spelt can absorb the liquid.

Noon: Fruit as your raw food; warm spelt with milk, sour milk, or buttermilk; or boiled potatoes with yogurt cheese (enrich with flaxseed oil to taste)

Afternoon: Drink plenty of fluids, but choose tea rather than water.

Evening: Potato vegetable soup (see p. 79 for recipe, with larger pieces of potatoes and vegetables) or home-fried potatoes with raw sauerkraut

Recommendation 3: A Variety of Balanced Whole Foods

In this dietary option (which provides 1,000 to 1,500 calories per day), you rely completely on whole food ingredients (see also pp. 94–95). You will supply your body not only with essential proteins, carbohydrates, and fat but also with all the valuable vitamins, minerals, trace elements, and other micronutrients it requires to stay healthy and fit. Highly nutritious whole food satisfies longer and, thanks to its high dietary fiber content, it stimulates digestion naturally. Moreover, with this diet option you do not consume a single unnecessary calorie—provided, of course, that you enjoy these foods in moderation. In any event, continue to drink plenty of fluids—but always between your meals, not with them.

HEALTHY NOURISHMENT
Rely on fresh fruits and vegetables. Dietary supplements can never replace the nourishment that high-quality foods provide to our bodies, because our bodies do not process these nutrients in isolation nearly as well as they do in nature's own combinations.

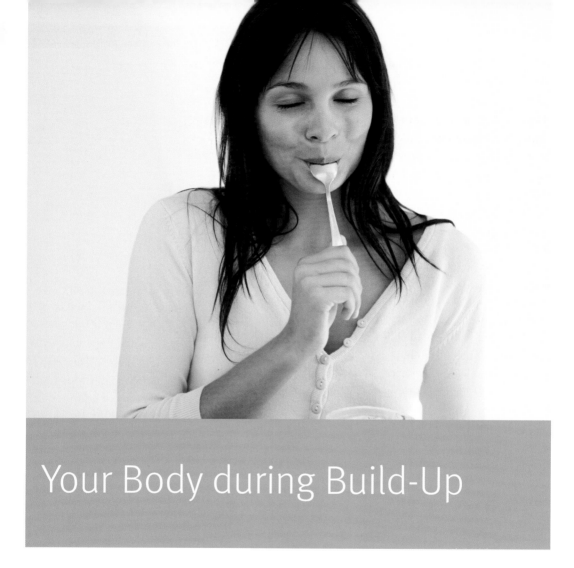

Your Body during Build-Up

It cannot be repeated often enough: even though this seems counterintuitive, the dietary build-up period after your fast is actually far more important than the fast itself. Moreover, it demands the same prerequisites as the fast, that is, peace of mind and a sense that you are protected, safe, and not rushed. Accordingly, at least one third of the length of the fasting time should be devoted to the dietary build-up period, because your body must slowly become accustomed to everyday life again and to the "task" of eating.

Digestive Juices

No digestive juices are produced during a fast, which is why you experience no hunger pangs. During the dietary build-up period these juices are initially produced in small quantities and then gradually in greater quantities. From your own "stomach sense," you can recognize how quickly and how much your gastric juices are beginning to flow again. This is why you should not simply eat whatever is placed in front of you. Instead, determine for yourself anew, every day and for every meal, how much you can tolerate and digest. The body that has been cleansed by fasting sends signals that will be recognized far more clearly than ever before.

> **"I am satisfied" means** "My hunger has been appeased. I don't need anything more. I'm going to stop eating [important!] and leave the rest on my plate."
> **"I am full" means** "My stomach is filled to capacity. It is more than I can digest. Half-digested food produces the uncomfortable sensation of being bloated and filled with gas; I don't feel well."
> **"I cannot eat any more" means** "My stomach is now stretched past capacity. I've exceeded my ability to digest it all."

The Cardiovascular System

Approximately one third of all the work performed by our cardiovascular system is needed for managing digestion. This third was unused during our fasting period. So do not be surprised if your physical performance declines somewhat during the first two build-up days. You might feel tired more often than usual, or find that you feel dizzy or as if your head is empty. After mealtime in particular a large amount of blood flows into the abdominal area—blood that is no longer available to the head or the muscles.

To aid the body, lie down after every meal (at noontime, in bed if possible). Before you get up, tense your muscles; extend your limbs and stretch, first tightening your muscles and then relaxing them. Do not make any exaggerated movements. Continue to drink ample amounts of fluids: 1½ to 2 quarts (1.5 to 2 L) of water, tea, or fruit juice diluted with carbonated water per day.

SUPPORTING DIGESTION

> Vigorous chewing, raw fruits and vegetables, fruit acids (raw apples), lactic acid (sour milk, yogurt), and aromatic herbs stimulate the production of gastric juices.
> Hurrying and hectic activity, cold feet, irritation, and ice-cold foods inhibit the production of gastric juices.

Water Balance

After the fast your body absorbs up to 1 quart (1 L) of water during the three dietary build-up days. This water is needed for the production of gastric juices and to keep the mucous membranes moist. The water also helps to balance the cardiovascular system, which will be fully stabilized no later than the third day of dietary build-up. Furthermore, the water also creates better internal tension for all the cells of the body, which in turn is evident through the tightening up of the complexion and the disappearance of small wrinkles.

Naturally, this additional fluid will show up on the scale. Even if you are disappointed with this additional weight, remember that any artificial elimination of this "operating fluid" by using diuretics is both absurd and dangerous. Continue to drink more than your thirst demands in between meals, just as you did during your fast. Be sure to drink sufficient amounts of fluid to ensure soft and voluminous stools. This will help greatly in maintaining your new weight.

THE ALPHA AND THE OMEGA—LIVELY BOWEL ACTION

The following promote normal evacuation of the bowels:

> Mornings, on an empty stomach, 1 glass water (warm for irritable bowels, cold for constipated bowels) or ½ glass water mixed with ½ glass sauerkraut juice
> Softened prunes, figs, or Bircher muesli (see p. 84 for the recipe)
> Fiber-rich foods (flaxseeds, raw fruits and vegetables, whole-grain bread, whole-grain cereal, wheat bran), always chewed thoroughly
> 1 ½ to 2 quarts (1.5 to 2 L) water or a similar liquid per day
> Physical activity of any kind
> Time and quiet for a bowel movement

These are things that inhibit the normal evacuation of the bowels:

> Getting up late
> Inactivity in any form
> A sedentary occupation with no compensating activity
> Hectic activity, time pressures, stress
> Cold hands or cold feet
> Insufficient hydration
> Impatient clenching and pushing

Give your body some time, even if you have suffered from constipation for years. And never give up.

Bowel Functions

The first independent evacuation of the bowels will take place on the second or often even the third dietary build-up day, because the bowels become activated only when they are filled. So be patient. To make things go a little more quickly, you should treat your intestines to roughage and stool softeners (dietary fiber). They will make you feel full and satisfied and will aid in the elimination process. The following are the best roughage and softeners:

> Flaxseeds: 2 teaspoons at every meal (take with plenty of fluid)
> Generous quantities of raw foods, such as fruits, vegetables, and salad
> Whole-grain bread or whole-grain cereal
> Plenty of liquid, preferably water or unsweetened teas

One problem during the dietary build-up period: often the rectum is still blocked by the somewhat dry stool formed during the fast. You sense that the intestines are moving, but the anus will not open. In this case there are methods that do not disrupt the entire gastrointestinal tract but instead affect only the rectum:

> Enema with 3½ fluid ounces (100 mL) warm water (enema syringe)
> A small enema with ½ quart (0.5 L) water
> Glycerin suppository (from the drugstore)

These measures are necessary for as long as there are problems with elimination. If you tend to be constipated, learn the basic principles for better gastric motility (see previous box).

Dealing with Postfast Discomfort

Like the fast, the first two dietary build-up days can introduce a flare-up of symptoms that existed before the fast. Everything usually gets straightened out again by the next day, though. Because the question of what fasting achieves can be answered only at the end of the dietary build-up period, be sure not to draw your final conclusions prematurely.

IMPORTANT

Every bite of food that is not well chewed or is superfluous causes bloating, because you also swallow air when you eat your food hastily.

TIP FOR SUCCESS

If you suffer from flatulence and distension, these gentle home remedies can eliminate the air from the gastrointestinal system:

> Warm moist compress with a hot water bottle (liver compress, see p. 52) for people who have a tendency to chills
> Cold compress (Priessnitz compress, see p. 56) for people who tend to be excessively hot
> Caraway-fennel tea or "four winds tea" (a mixture of chamomile blossoms, peppermint leaves, caraway seeds, and fennel seeds, from the drugstore or the Internet)
> Purging the intestines with natural aids from the drugstore: enemas and glycerin suppositories

All too often, by the third or fourth day of dietary rebuilding the joie de vivre and ability to enjoy normal life we regain through fasting tempt us to go overboard. What happens then is perhaps best illustrated by the experiences a group of fasters candidly described before they left a clinic.

Three men and two women who became acquainted during their fast at the clinic and spent a lot of time together decided to celebrate the end of their fast. After the first dietary build-up day they agreed to meet at a nice restaurant for an ample farewell meal together.

Case One

Even during his fast, Mr. W. dreamed of a big steak. He gobbled it down greedily without leaving anything on his plate. Three hours later, back at the fasting clinic, he rang for the night nurse because of terrible abdominal cramps. "I could not live and I could not die" is how he described his condition. Only after he vomited the remnants of his half-digested food was he finally able to sink back into his bed, deathly pale and drenched in sweat but relieved of his pain.

Reason: In the process of decomposition, undigested protein (present in especially high volumes in meat) generates by-products that act like a poison to the sensitized body.

Case Two

Ms. S., who had lost 3 pounds during her fast, allowed herself a complete meal, with ice cream topped with whipped cream as the crowning final indulgence. That evening her distended stomach made it all too clear that this did not agree with her. Even worse, however, was that the next morning her scale registered a weight gain of almost 3 pounds (1.3 kg)—three days of fasting for nothing.

Reason: during this very sensitive postfast period every little extra calorie sticks with you.

Case Three

Mr. A. spent too much time at the restaurant drinking good wine. Late that night his friends had to carry him home and put him to bed. The laboratory report revealed what had happened: his liver function levels had jumped precipitously.

Reason: just as during the fast, during the dietary build-up period the liver takes a little "vacation," and its tolerance for alcohol is significantly reduced. Even small quantities can make you inebriated and damage the liver cells.

Case Four

Ms. K. had eaten modestly but ordered a cup of coffee to end the meal. Later she was surprised that the night seemed as if it would never end. She lay wide awake in bed, pondering to herself, "But I've always been able to sleep well after a cup of coffee in the evening. What's wrong with me?"

Reason: after a fast the nervous system reacts much more sensitively to stimulants of all kinds—coffee as well as medications.

Case Five

Mr. N. ordered only an easily digestible fish dinner. Surprisingly, soon he felt satisfied and so he left half his portion on the plate. He suffered from no complaints. He had truly wanted to follow the guidelines for the dietary build-up period to the letter, however, so why in the world (he wondered) had he let the others talk him into going along to the restaurant?

During the fast the group had been good-natured and ready to have fun. Why did everything go so badly at the grand good-bye celebration? During the entire fast, while drinking only water, they managed to dance and have a good time with each other. Why did their celebration fail? Was it because eating and drinking were now the focus?

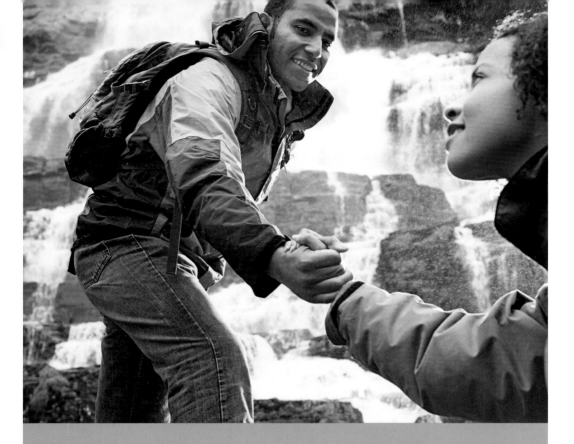

Sustaining the Benefits of Your Fast

How are things progressing in your daily life now? During the fast and the dietary build-up period you had many experiences. Now take the bull by the horns and use this opportunity to break the vicious cycle of bad dietary and poor living habits. After all, in recent days you recognized that you were succeeding, regardless of whether you had given up smoking or some other unhealthy habit. You sensed that you do have the power to turn your life in another direction. Take advantage of this:

> Take a piece of paper and write down what you would like to change. Be sure to take stock while you are still in your fasting and dietary build-up period.
> For the coming weeks set up a nutritional program and a schedule for the kind of exercise that suits you best, one that you can actually achieve in the framework of your daily life.
> In the future do without nicotine, alcohol, and other noxious substances (e.g., coffee) as much as possible.
> Participate in the creation of self-help groups. Share your experiences and also help others.

A Practice That Makes You Stronger

Take advantage of your new awareness that your body can do without food completely from time to time and that when doing so you can nonetheless feel good and be fit.

> Skip meals when you have no appetite for them. You will discover that you do not need them and do not even miss them.
> Often your body can answer the question "Am I full?" only after waiting 10 minutes after eating. Allow it that time.
> Fast when you have a fever, diarrhea, or indigestion. Your body will thank you for it.

Make firm plans for your next fast now, perhaps together with your friends.

Find Your Balance

Continue with what you learned in your gradual build-up of food. You may eat what you wish as long as you can rely on the signals from your body: "When I am full, I will stop." Do this and you will never need calorie tables or nutritional charts; you will need only a scale.

Most people, however, do not trust the physical sensations of their own bodies and feel more secure following instructions. If this describes you, look for a good book on wholesome cooking, as well as other nutritional guidebooks that can be of help (see p. 112).

ANOTHER FAST
Repeat the fasting week as soon as you have the time and opportunity in your job or your private life. Your second or third fast will be easier than the first. Each fast is different and brings interesting new experiences. People who can maintain their weight in the meantime will be able to lose weight gradually with several short fasts throughout the year.

One Preparation Day Each Week

After you have fasted, 800 or 1,000 calories per day will seem ample to you. You will feel full quickly, and you will also feel satisfied. These apparently modest quantities of food will be sufficient because, despite your low caloric intake, these smaller quantities contain everything your body needs. Anyone who cannot manage over the long term with such low-calorie, high-nutritional-quality food should recall the Preparation Day that introduced their fast:

> Get in the regular habit of introducing a fruit day, rice day, or fresh vegetable day once a week (see p. 34)—for example, every Monday or Friday, or maybe even both days. The important thing is for you to develop your preparation days into a new habit.

Steps Toward a Whole-Food Diet

The most common diseases of our times are partly caused by poor nutrition. Quantitatively we are overfed, but qualitatively we are undernourished. In concrete terms this means that we eat too much, but unfortunately much of what we eat is nutritionally inferior. Our diets are characterized by fatty and sugar-rich foodstuffs that provide little to no nutritional value for our bodies. Our bodies, however, must nevertheless process these foodstuffs, and so it stores them in deposits that collect around the hips, stomach, and buttocks. It has long been apparent that diet pills and shots can do nothing to help. For anyone who recognizes this fact, there is only one solution: a change in diet.

Eating Whole Foods in Everyday Life

Fasting creates a break in old nutritional habits. The switch that previously seemed so difficult is easier to accomplish after a fast. It is not necessary to change everything at once; you can approach it step by step, but by all means make some changes to your nutritional habits. Nutritionists Werner Kollath and Herbert Warning coined a formula that everyone can live by:

EAT AS NEEDED

Are you someone who is often hungry? Then you are doing the right thing if you eat five or six times a day—small meals that you chew slowly and thoroughly.

w	v	m	l
Wholesome	Varied	Moderate	Lean

Regardless of your daily life, think about your past dietary habits and have the courage to start to nourish yourself with nutritious whole food every day. On the following pages you will find 12 Golden Rules to help you to change your diet gradually.

Whole-grain noodles, fresh fruits and vegetables, flavorful herbs, and high-quality vegetable oil—these are only a little foretaste of what whole-food cuisine has to offer.

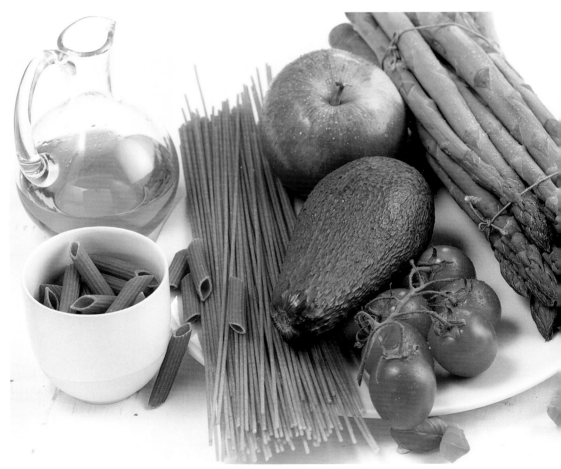

The 12 Simple Rules

1. Use whole-grain bread instead of white bread.
Replace white bread and rolls with whole-grain bread, which makes you feel full more quickly and for a longer period. Virtually all varieties of bread can be made from whole grains, either freshly cracked or ground fine, from flatbread to coarse-grained bread, and even whole-grain rolls.

2. Use whole-grain flour.
Choose whole-grain flour rather than white flour when you bake and cook, and remember that it is best when freshly ground. The bran from the whole grain contains many valuable ingredients, such as vitamins, minerals, nutrition-rich oils, and proteins.

3. Eat raw fruits and vegetables before the meal.
Cooking destroys most beneficial plant nutrients. In their raw form, fruits and vegetables contain all valuable vitamins, enzymes, and minerals in natural bindings. An additional advantage is that raw fruits and vegetables pass through the stomach more quickly.

4. Limit the amounts of sugar and sweets.
Jams, chocolate, cake, cookies, sodas, and ice cream have no nutritional value. Eaten often and in excess, they make you fat, destroy your teeth, and ruin your health. Sweeten your food sparingly with honey or with apple or pear syrup. Softened dates, figs, and dried bananas are also good as sweeteners. Persons with diabetes and overweight people should use artificial sweeteners.

5. Use small amounts of salt.
We take in far too much salt. It binds water in the body, promotes high blood pressure, and stresses the heart and kidneys. Season your food using fresh or dried herbs instead. Moreover, highly nutritional whole food has spice and flavor of its own. Give your sense of taste the chance to recognize this and to savor the variety of these foods.

6. Use fat sparingly.
Watch out for hidden fats in particular, and buy only lean cold cuts and cheeses. In the kitchen, use cold-pressed vegetable oils when possible; they provide the body with many nutritionally valuable substances.

7. Use animal proteins sparingly.

The body needs proteins from a variety of sources. In the case of a mixed whole-food diet the correct proportion is two thirds vegetable protein (e.g., grain) and one third animal protein from milk products, eggs, meat, and fish. For a vegetarian whole-food diet the proportion is two thirds from plants and grains and one third from dairy products, eggs, soy, yeast, and nuts.

8. Pay attention to the proper balance.

Your daily nutritional intake should be made up of 12 to 15 percent protein, 30 to 35 percent high-nutritional fats, and 50 to 60 percent carbohydrates.

9. Choose your beverages wisely.

What the body really needs is pure, clear water in between mealtimes. Diluted fruit juices, as well as herbal teas you have prepared yourself, provide some variety. Milk is actually liquid food, and its caloric and protein contents must be taken into account. Coffee and black tea should be drunk only by those who need a pick-me-up, because both of these beverages are stimulants. Wine, beer, and spirits are beverages consumed for their taste or effects and are intoxicants, thus totally unsuited to satisfying thirst; they are also high in calories.

10. Value quality before quantity.

When you are shopping, focus on foods with high nutritional value. Certified organic fruits and vegetables are not only healthier and better for you, they also keep longer than foods grown with artificial fertilizers and treated with chemicals. Meat, poultry, and eggs produced in accordance with natural and animal-friendly farming practices are more expensive, yet you will need less of them to feel full.

11. Choose items that are as natural as possible.

Pay attention to the additives in products (coloring, flavorings, and preservatives). Whatever you need should be prepared with as little processing as possible.

12. Choose items that are as fresh as possible.

There should be minimal time between harvest, purchase, preparation, and consumption. This is especially true for fresh juices and fresh raw fruits and vegetables, which lose food value and flavor if they stand even for half an hour. Fresh and frozen vegetables have more nutritional value than canned vegetables.

Fasting: A Time for Reflection

The fasting experience can touch the deeper layers of the human being because it is a time when you are confronted with your own self more intensely than in your normal day-to-day existence. Fasting is a time for contemplation.

Virtually all people who fast report that, along with the purely physical experience they gain through the fast, which is primarily focused on eating, drinking, and pleasurable behavior, they achieve other multifaceted spiritual insights. Even in your first exposure to fasting, you too will appreciate that it can be the path to inner freedom and independence in both thought and action.

The profundity of the meaning of fasting and the full range of its healing effects, though, can be explored only in lengthy or repeated fasts. If the experience of this week of fasting has encouraged you to undertake a longer fast, then the purpose of this book has been fulfilled.

Preventive Fasting

Everyone should have the experience of fasting at least once in his or her lifetime. Learning that we can live without nourishment for a time, and then eat more modestly than usual, is in itself a valuable experience. It is recommended that every healthy person from the age of 30 onward should fast occasionally. The so-called fasting weeks for healthy people have proved their value. Under expert direction, people get together in their hometowns or on vacation to fast together. (This is quite popular in Europe and is just becoming better known in the United States.)

In light of our modern lifestyle, however, a general physical "overhaul" is advisable, and perhaps even necessary, by age 40 at the latest. In addition to permanent moderate conditioning training to maintain health and fitness, this should also include an "oil change" through a longer fast in an appropriate fasting clinic.

Prevention Is Better than a Cure

The most progressive health insurance plans have already recognized that it is less expensive to prevent diseases before they develop, by appropriate preventive measures, than it is to treat these illnesses at a later stage (which is often a much longer process). For this reason such plans are willing to help cover various early preventive measures, sometimes for up to three weeks. In this way they help the insured person experience a beneficial learning process, one that will pay off for the insurance companies in the future.

Prevention of What?

Anyone who wants to get fit and healthier can hardly find a better means to accomplish this than fasting. For example, a preventive fast against cancer (to the extent that you do not have a genetic predisposition) or for premature aging (arteriosclerosis) is most sensible. In addition, anyone who is overweight should fast, and not just for weight correction or weight control. From a fast, people can also learn how to manage their own predispositions and eating habits better.

EXCELLENT PROSPECTS
Often simply a glance at the scale is enough to reinforce the desire for the success of a fast. Not only does personal well-being increase with every pound lost, but personal health also benefits.

WHO SHOULD FAST?

Anyone with an elevated risk of illness from diet-induced health problems or metabolic stress should fast at regular intervals, that is, as long as it takes to eliminate the risk factors that can be tracked by laboratory tests.

The positive effects of fasting on high-risk symptoms are apparent in the following cases:

> Tendency to high blood pressure (hypertension)
> Blood lipid levels too high (elevated cholesterol and triglyceride levels)
> Elevated blood sugar (prediabetes)
> Overproduction of blood cells and excessively thick blood (polycythemia)
> Elevated uric acid level in the blood (the early stages of gout)

The following example illustrates how determined people can be in modifying their eating and drinking habits after fasting, thereby influencing their body weight.

A man 43 years of age and 5 feet 7 inches (166 cm) tall weighed in at about 200 pounds (91 kg)—or 40 percent overweight—at the beginning of his fast. Over the course of four years, during which he undertook four fasting cures, he decreased his weight to 154 pounds (70 kg)—or 10 percent overweight.

> Year 1, after 15 fast days: Lost 24 lb. (11 kg)
> Year 2, after 18 fast days: Lost 19 lb. (8.5 kg)
> Year 3, after 11 fast days: Lost 15 lb. (6.8 kg)
> Year 4, after 11 fast days: Lost 13½ lb. (6.2 kg)

In total, this meant not only a loss of nearly 71 pounds (20 kg) but also the lowering of five risk factors that can lead to serious diseases (see box on p. 99). Even more important, however, the man gained an increased sense of well-being that cannot be measured on any scale.

Take Your Time

"Slowly but surely" is the old saying (think of the fable of the tortoise and the hare), if you would like to reduce your personal risk of disease with the aid of fasting. After all, it is not possible to lose in a few days or even a few weeks what you have gained over the course of a lifetime. You should plan on gradual weight loss through several fasts and reductions in weight. Keep your goal in sight, even during those periods when you are not fasting. Always be thinking about complete, light, whole-food nutrition.

ARE YOU OVERWEIGHT?

A clear indicator that you should lose weight for health reasons is your waist measurement. Place a measuring tape between your lower costal arch and the crest of your ilium at the largest point of your abdomen. For men the measurement should not exceed 37 inches (94 cm), and for women it should be no more than 31½ inches (80 cm), regardless of height.

What about Alcohol and Nicotine?

Have You Wanted to Give Up Smoking for a Long Time? Did You Notice That Fasting Is One of the More Effective Aids in Quitting?

The flavor of a cigarette has also been changed by your sense of taste, which was heightened through your fast. Often it will taste like straw—bland, sometimes even disgusting. Why are you smoking, anyway? After having quit smoking during your fast, you know that you can indeed follow through on your decision. Basically, your smoking cessation training has already begun.

In the same way, you also proved to yourself during your fast that you can do without alcohol. The break in drinking was good for your liver, but it was also important for your self-confidence. Anyone who is accustomed to drinking alcohol regularly is constantly in danger of slipping unconsciously into dependency. After not drinking alcohol for a week, you are now strong enough to review your relationship with alcohol. If your fasting week gave you any indication that some form of dependency exists, you should not hesitate to contact Alcoholics Anonymous (AA), groups of people nationwide with similar experiences who support each other in their resolve not to drink. Fasting and friends provide a new impetus to overcome this dependency.

Self-Help Groups

Regardless of whether it be eating, drinking, smoking, or some other life experience, the isolated person always finds it more difficult to succeed than a group pursuing the same goals. If you want to manage your tendency to overeat, seek out others with the same problem. In the United States, Overeaters Anonymous (OA) and Weight Watchers can help you attain success.

Share Your Experience!

Invite other fasters to join you and share your experiences. Deeper conversations develop naturally; if you have the courage to discuss your own problems, this will encourage others to open up too. Do not escape into typical meaningless small talk. You might discover that you are not the only one with problems.

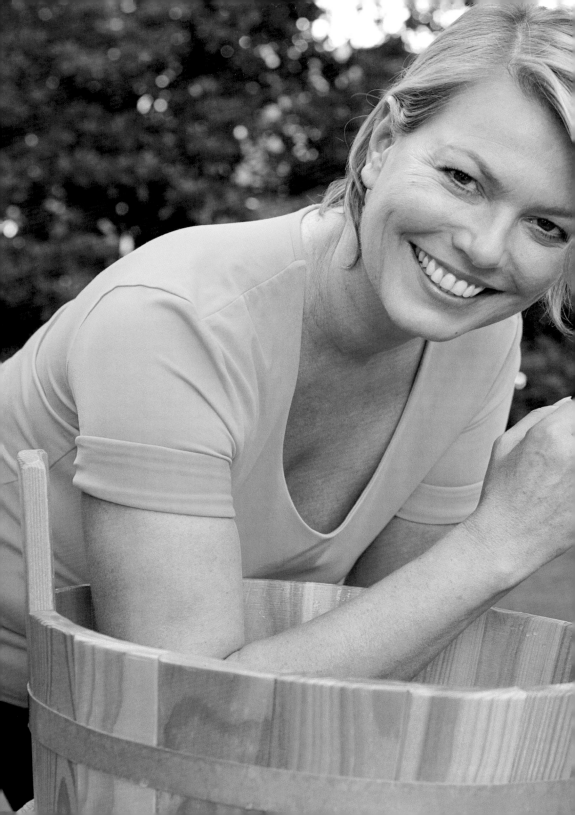

THERAPEUTIC FASTING

Extended therapeutic fasts are conducted under medical supervision at a fasting clinic, where you will also learn how to change your previous dietary and lifestyle habits. This chapter is written from the European perspective, as fasting there has been a part of the healing repertoire for such a long period of time.

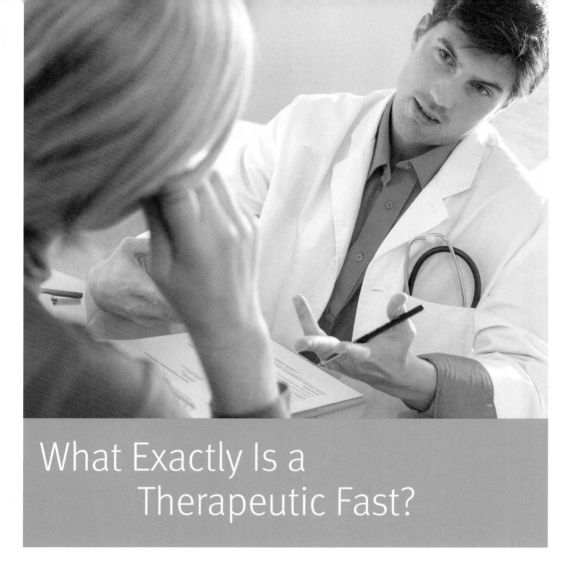

What Exactly Is a Therapeutic Fast?

Therapeutic fasting is a form of natural medicine, which unfortunately is not as widely known as it should be, despite the fact that it has proved itself to be an extremely effective method of treatment. This is especially true for diet-induced metabolic disorders and their often extremely serious consequences. Preventive or precautionary measures can also be considered healing treatments when they help to quickly and effectively eliminate the precursors to life-threatening illnesses. In this way, starting as early as possible, you can do your part to prevent heart attacks, strokes, and cerebral or peripheral vascular disease. With a great deal of patience you could also achieve this same goal through long-term dietary changes and regular exercise. But, in all honesty, who can manage that—particularly when you are busy with your everyday professional life? Is there really anyone willing to make these fundamental lifestyle changes in a daily routine that often has become quite comfortable?

Nothing can encourage a person's will and inner strength for change more effectively than a fast. Therapeutic fasting is the only way not just to eliminate dangerous risk factors quickly but also to show persons at risk that they can succeed in rectifying bad dietary habits and live without alcohol or tobacco in the long run. The rule is this: the more serious the health risk, the heavier the dependence on previous consumption habits, the more threatening the disease, the longer the therapeutic fast and the accompanying dietary and behavioral training should last. It is understandable that few people can achieve this on their own. For this reason persons wanting to significantly improve their health are urged to stay at least three to four weeks at a fasting clinic with a specially trained staff.

COMPETENT CARE

Intensive group and individual discussions, diabetic counseling, and a teaching kitchen, as well as progressive movement therapy, are the methods used by the specialists at a fasting clinic to achieve permanent changes in their patients' behavior.

About Costs and Benefits

By now you are probably asking yourself, "How much does [preventive] treatment like this cost?" Here's a sample case.

A 43-year-old mechanic has suffered from diabetes for a decade. As a result of this disease he developed severe ulcers on the soles of both his feet, which after a year led to his being unable to work. Although his skin was treated with care and his blood glucose levels were adjusted with medication, the ulcers on his feet did not improve. Only after a 21-day therapeutic fast in a clinic, the change to a whole-food diet rich in vital nutrients, and a newly adjusted diabetes management plan did the ulcers on his feet heal within four weeks. The patient was able to return to work as before.

Two years later the patient returned to the clinic; his successful cure had lasted just one year. The reason for his visit was his dramatic weight gain. The patient's lifestyle and therefore his diabetes, too, were now totally out of control. Furthermore, the ulcers on the soles of his feet had reappeared. This time they were meticulously treated with a special diet, insulin, and modern medications at a university clinic. In addition to the physical strain brought on by such treatment, the patient was once again unable to work for another year. The cost of his diabetes treatment was amounting to about $20,500.

Another therapeutic fast of 21 days, followed by a reintroduction period, resulted in a weight loss of 31 pounds (14 kg). His elevated blood lipid levels went down, the thickening of his blood (polyglobulism) was reduced, and his blood sugar levels were normalized, even without the use of insulin and other medications. Even the ulcers on his feet healed completely. Because of the changes in his diet and diabetes medication, the man was doing so well that he was able to accept an installation job

PAYMENT OPTIONS FOR FASTING TREATMENT*

> The patient is a *direct payer*. Most fasting clinics are private clinics; partial reimbursement by health insurance is possible, but you should ask your insurance company
> Subsidy by health insurance for treatment at a specialized clinic
> Full reimbursement by the insurer, as would be the case for a hospital stay
> Partial reimbursement from government assistance

The more serious the illness and the more successfully it can be treated through an inpatient therapeutic fast at a clinic, the more willing a health insurance company is to make a correspondingly greater investment. Experience has shown that hospital treatment of diet-induced metabolic disorders is significantly more expensive than inpatient therapeutic fasts at a specialized clinic, which in most cases show better results. Many health insurance plans are now favorably disposed toward financing inpatient preventive treatments if diseases can be prevented.

* *This information was originally provided for German readers. Fasting is a new practice in the United States. Insurance companies will develop their own approach over time.*

abroad. Restaurant meals and the boredom of empty evenings far from home proved a disastrous combination for him, however, leading to another period of weight gain. Once again his diabetes slipped out of control, and with it his entire metabolism. This resulted in deposits in the tiniest blood vessels (capillaries), especially in his feet. The thickened blood flowed more slowly, impairing blood circulation, and the ulcers did not heal. The result? Another nine months on disability and additional medical costs of about $26,000.

The third therapeutic fast (25 days, followed by a 15-day nutritional training session) once again effected a cure. The disrupted metabolism was corrected, the blood thinned, and the pathologic changes in the capillaries were eliminated. What other medical treatment could accomplish this? A few weeks at a fasting clinic yielded this result for about $4,100—a fraction of the costs incurred by the other treatment methods, not to mention lost work time and income.

ALLERGIC REACTIONS

With allergic and rheumatic diseases a lengthy abstention from food and the stimulation of all natural excretions can cause a modification in the body's mode of reacting (desensitization) and can initiate a change in the immune system, thereby commencing the healing process. There are astounding possibilities here, but remember this: all these positive changes can occur only in a body that is still responsive. If the disease is already advanced (as in chronic illness), the attempt is often not very successful.

Fasting: A Radical Method

Therapeutic fasting is a thousand-year-old remedy. In contrast to many other treatment methods, it gets to the roots of the disease and personal behavior. In the hands of an experienced fasting doctor at a fasting clinic, it is a safe yet effective treatment method. It obeys natural laws that are grounded in the nature of human beings. Scientific proof for it has existed in the medical community for a long time. A lengthy fast of 18, 24, or 32 days or even longer has a profound effect on the metabolic processes of the afflicted person. This "operation without a scalpel" offers significant advantages over surgical intervention: it harms nothing, yet at the same time it reaches down into every cell in every organ, every tiny capillary, and remote recesses in the connective tissue where disease-inducing substances might have been deposited. Moreover, the patient is fully conscious of this type of intervention. In this way healing goes hand in hand with important insights and the patient's growing sense of well-being.

Candidates for a Stay at a Fasting Clinic

Therapeutic fasting is especially appropriate for diet-induced metabolic disorders, chronic illnesses, and diseases of the musculoskeletal system closely connected with metabolic imbalances. Many patients have several health challenges simultaneously, or in combination, that require an individual diagnosis. Therapeutic fasting can help with the following:

> Severe obesity (more than 30 percent overweight)
> Diabetes
> Gout
> Polyglobulism (overabundance of red blood cells)
> Fatty liver
> Chronic hepatitis (liver cell damage)
> Arterial circulatory disorders (e.g., coronary artery or peripheral vascular disease)
> Hypertension (high blood pressure)
> Elevated risk of a heart attack
> Rheumatic disorders requiring the elimination of toxins and readjustment of the reaction system, such as nonarticular rheumatism, rheumatoid arthritis, and cases of damage to the spinal disks and joints (e.g., spondylarthrosis, osteochondrosis, arthrosis)
> Chronic skin diseases (e.g., eczema, neurodermatitis, psoriasis)
> Venous circulatory disorders causing ulcerated legs
> Allergic disorders of the skin and mucous membranes

Even diseases that seem incurable or do not respond to treatment can be healed, or their progression can be halted, through fasting and natural complementary treatment. These diseases include the following:

> Migraines and chronic headaches

TIP

Everyone should get a regular comprehensive health checkup. Most health insurance plans cover annual or biannual exams. If you have health coverage, take advantage of this offer; it is a good opportunity to discover and treat personal risk factors by such measures as therapeutic fasting.

NORMALIZATION OF HIGH BLOOD PRESSURE AND WEIGHT REDUCTION AFTER A THREE-WEEK FAST

The diagram contains the average values for 215 overweight fasting patients (results of Dr. H. Fahrner).

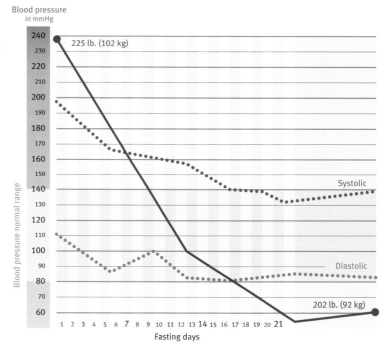

> Glaucoma in its early stages
> Porphyria, polyarthritis, Bechterew's disease (ankylosing spondylitis), Reiter's disease, and the early stages of Crohn's disease
  Last but not least, lengthy fasts can interrupt eating disorders and addictions and so, when used in combination with psychiatric therapy, can be a definite help with the following:
> Gluttony, sugar addiction, bulimia
> Propensity toward addiction to alcohol, nicotine, and prescription drugs

Who Should Not Fast?

Fasting is generally a positive experience for many people; still, not everyone can tolerate extended abstention from food. Fasting is not suitable for the following persons:

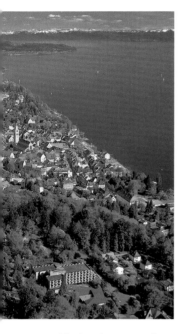

The lovely surroundings and pleasant atmosphere in Überlingen on Lake Constance ensure a successful fast at this clinic.

> People without reserves, that is, those who are poorly nourished or physically and emotionally exhausted (e.g., after a long illness or a serious operation); patients who suffer from pathological weight loss (e.g., in tuberculosis or cancer)

> People who are psychologically unstable because they cannot take responsibility for their own actions; under the supervision of a physician, though, good results have been observed in patients with schizophrenia and depression

> People who are under severe mental stress because they lack inner peace and a sense of security; in patients with neuroses, additional psychotherapeutic treatment is required (available at the fasting clinic)

> People who are overstressed mentally and physically (such people should first take eight days of vacation before they begin a lengthy fast)

> Patients who are being treated with Marcumar (phenprocoumon) or similar anticoagulants

Inpatient Fasting Treatment

An inpatient fasting treatment is a carefully planned therapeutic treatment of a predetermined duration of three, four, or more weeks under a physician's supervision. During the treatment the person fasting stays with other like-minded people at a spa or specialized clinic in an environment designed to support fasting. He or she submits voluntarily to strict house rules, which may prohibit alcohol and nicotine and ensure sufficient rest in the afternoon and at night. These rules, without exception, require conduct appropriate to therapeutic treatment. Adherence to these strict rules is amply compensated for by the indisputably pleasant ambiance, with its bright colors and a beautiful atmosphere that is a delight to the senses. The setting for a fast should not be like a hospital.

Providing a Getaway from Your Daily Routine

A certain fasting style has emerged from the long history of fasting clinics, especially in Germany, with its long and rich fasting tradition. It is a meaningful combination of fasting and post-fast diet, with the opportunity for customized physical activity including hiking, swimming, sports, and gymnastics. A successful stay at a fasting clinic also provides a connection with the natural environment—bracing light, fresh air, and water—amid a scenic landscape. The prescribed athletic activities and the stress-reducing environment are complemented with massages, baths, sauna, Kneipp treatments, and breathing and movement training. Personal growth is supported by diverse forms of health education in lectures, small-group projects, and the teaching kitchen. Music, conversations, and discussions round out the offerings. In addition to the previously described basic care for the participant in a preventive fast, the patient at a fasting clinic receives medical care comparable to that in a good hospital. Knowing this, you can understand why a "zero diet"—which is simply going without food—is not the same as a therapeutic fast, according to Dr. Otto Buchinger, even though both are forms of therapeutic abstention from food.

Success and a Stay at a Fasting Clinic

Inpatient therapeutic fasting at a fasting clinic is a scientifically based method of treatment under the supervision of experienced fasting doctors. The fasting clinic offers safety through modern diagnostic methods and progress observation by means of laboratory and cardiovascular tests. Doctors and nurses, just like their counterparts in regular hospitals, are on call 24 hours a day. Naturally, a therapeutic fast also includes the treatment plan, medical history, and other information provided to your primary care physician and health insurance provider. What is critical to the success of a lengthy fast at the clinic is good psychological care by a staff with experience in fasting, starting with the doctors, nurses, and participating therapists.

APPLYING FOR THERAPEUTIC TREATMENT

Discuss your desire for a therapeutic fast with your primary care physician. He or she will support your application for clinical inpatient treatment to your health insurance plan and will substantiate the medical grounds for the fast. In addition, you should contact a fasting clinic. Find out about the assistance you can expect from your health insurance. Health insurance plans may require documentation by a physician and the clinic.

Resources

Fasting

Brantschen, Nikolaus, *Fasting: What, Why, How.* ISBN978-0-824525408

Autogenic Training

Kermani, Kai. *Autogenic Training: The Effective Holistic Way to Better Health.*
ISBN 978-0285633223

Therapeutic Fasting Clinics in Germany

Buchinger-Klinik at Lake Constance has an international clientele and offers programs in
English (*http://www.buchinger.com*).
Kurpark-Klinik (more affordable) also at Lake Constance, can accommodate English guests
(*http://kurpark-klinik.de*).
Immanuel Krankenhaus Berlin (*http://www.immanuel.de*)

Other houses

The Clinic Dr. Otto Buchinger in Bad Pyrmont, Germany (*http://www.buchinger.de/lang-en*)
Die Malteser Klinik von Weckbecker in Bad Brückenau, Germany
(*http://www.weckbecker.com*)
Habichtswald-Klinik in Kassel, Germany (*http://www.habichtswaldklinik.de*)
Der Tannerhof in Bayrischzell, Germany (*http://www.tannerhof.de*)
Menschels Vitalresort in Meddersheim, Bad Sobernheim, Germany
(*http://www.menschel.com*)

To become a Certified Fasting Coach

Der Berufsverband Fasten und Ernährung e.V. (*http://www.bv-fasten-ernaehrung.de*)
Deutsche Fastenakademie e.V. (*http://www.d-f-a.de*)

Fasting Houses for People in Good Health

Landhaus Schiffmann (*http://www.landhaus-schiffmann.de*)
Landhaus Alger am See (*http://www.alger-fasten.de*)
Fastenwandern, Victoria and Dr. Helmut Zorn (*vhzorn@t-online.de*)
Kloster Pernegg (*http://www.klosterpernegg.at*)

Glauber's Salt

(Sal Mirabilis; $Na_2SO_410H_2O$) is a strong laxative; it is also used for dyeing, so
make sure that you buy Glauber's salt that is made for consumption, e.g. from
http://www.somaluna.com/prod/mirabilitum_glaubers_salt.asp

Reading Notes

Notes for Preparation Day

Notes for the First Day of Fasting

Notes for the Third Day of Fasting

Notes for Fifth Day of Fasting

Notes for the Second Build-Up Day

Masthead

ISBN 978-3-8338-0700-8

4th ed., 2009   1st edition 2008

Program Director: Ulrich Ehrlenspiel

Editor-in-Chief: Barbara Fellenberg

Editor: Sylvie Hinderberger

Photo Editor: Henrike Schechter

Layout: Independent Medien-Design, Claudia Hautkappe

Production: Petra Roth

Typesetting: Christopher Hammond

Reproduction: Repro Ludwig, Zell am See

Printing: Firmengruppe APPL, aprinta druck, Wemding

Binding: Firmengruppe APPL, sellier druck, Freising

Picture Credits:

Photo Production: STUDIO L'EVEQUE, Tanja & Harry Bischof

Graphics: Detlef Seidensticker

Additional Photos: Asia Pix: U2/p. 1; Corbis: pp. 54, 86; Digital Vision: pp. 30/31; Getty: pp. 6/7, 38, 76; GU: pp. 92 (L. Lenz), 95 (H. Bischof); Jump: pp. 3 right, 8, 20, 32, 74/75, 102/103; Photodisc: p. 44; Picturepress: U4 right; StockFood: U4 left.; Superbild: p. 104; H. von Waldersdorff: Cover

Important Notice

The thoughts, methods, and insights in this book represent the opinions and experience of the author. They were prepared and reviewed by the author with the greatest possible care. However, they do not replace competent, personal medical advice. Every reader remains responsible for his or her own acts and omissions. Neither the author nor the publisher can be held responsible for any loss or injury that may result from the practical guidance presented in this book.

Topical Index

Recipe Index